THE STORY OF CANCER
Volume 6

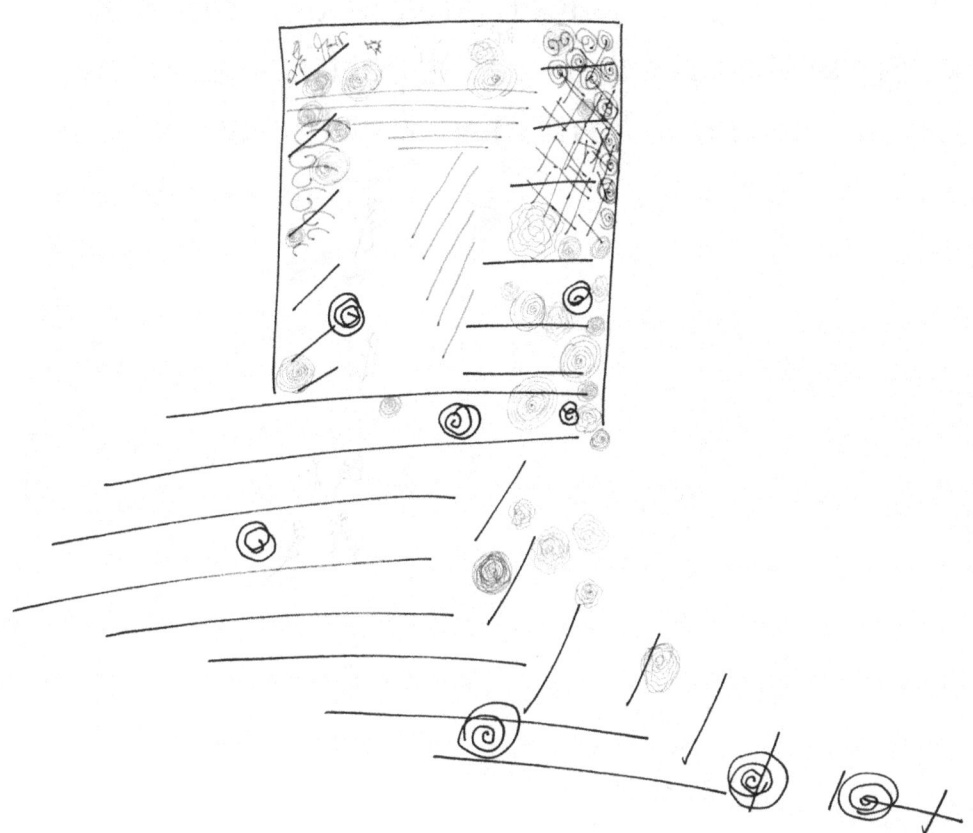

Camilia MacPherson, Ph.D., D.Th.
2016

INTRODUCTION

This is the Story of Cancer written using Automatic Drawings and Surreal Art. It is part of a continuous document written in 7 volumes.

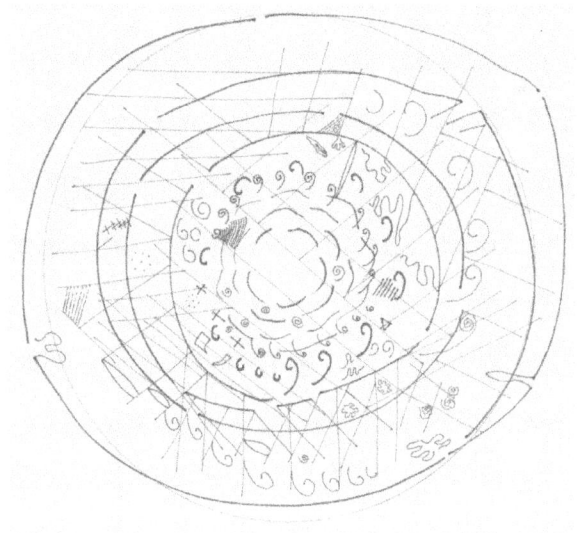

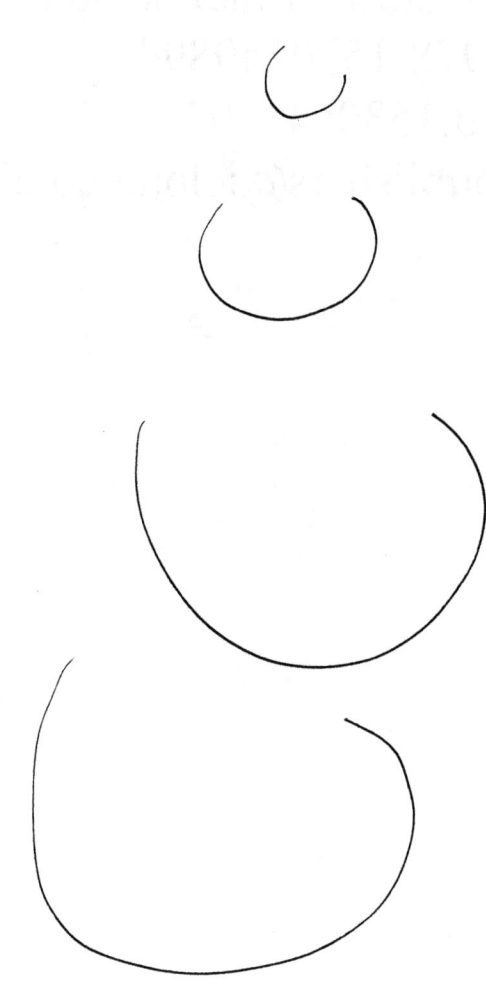

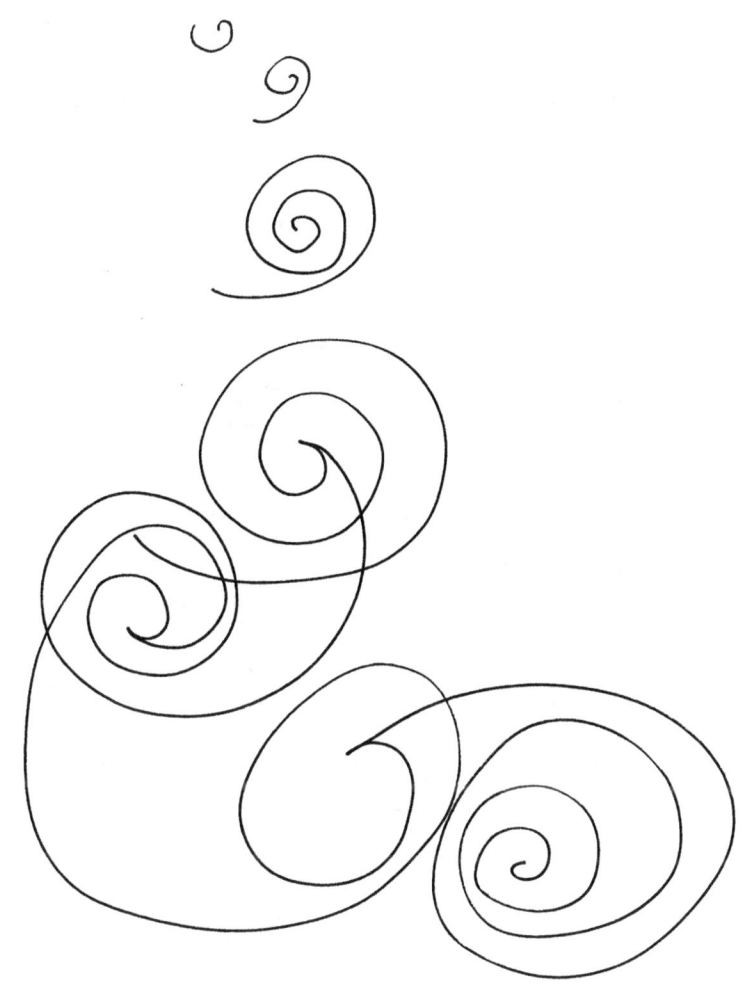

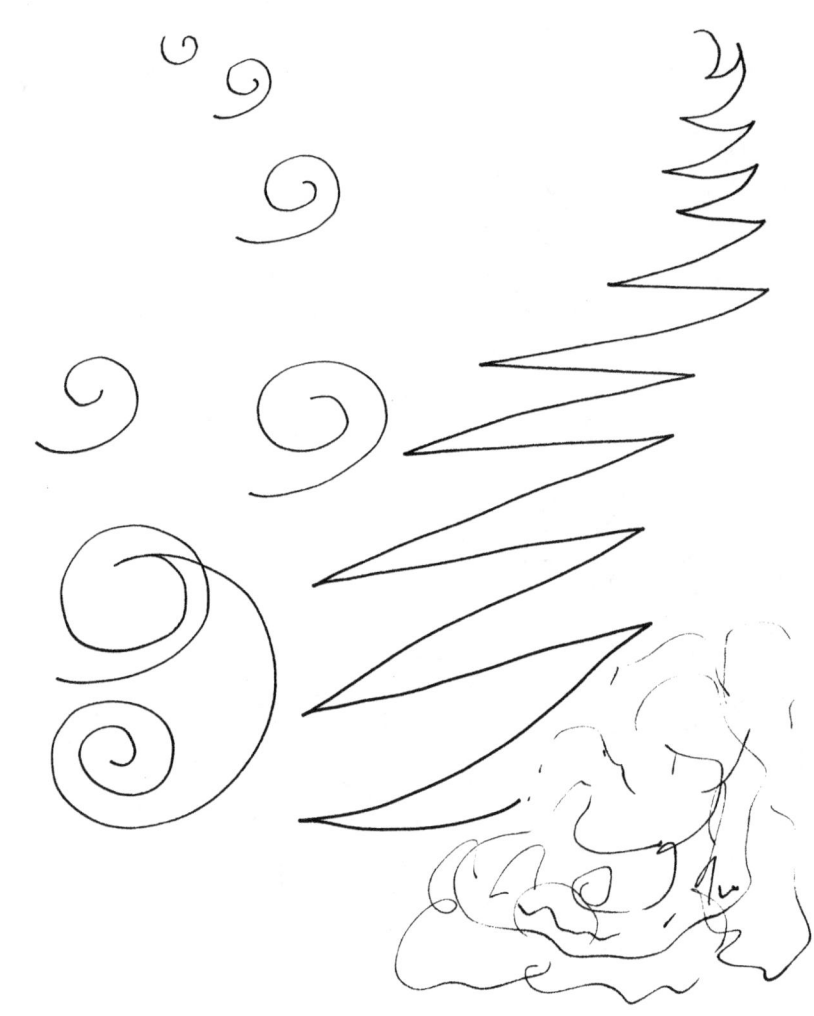

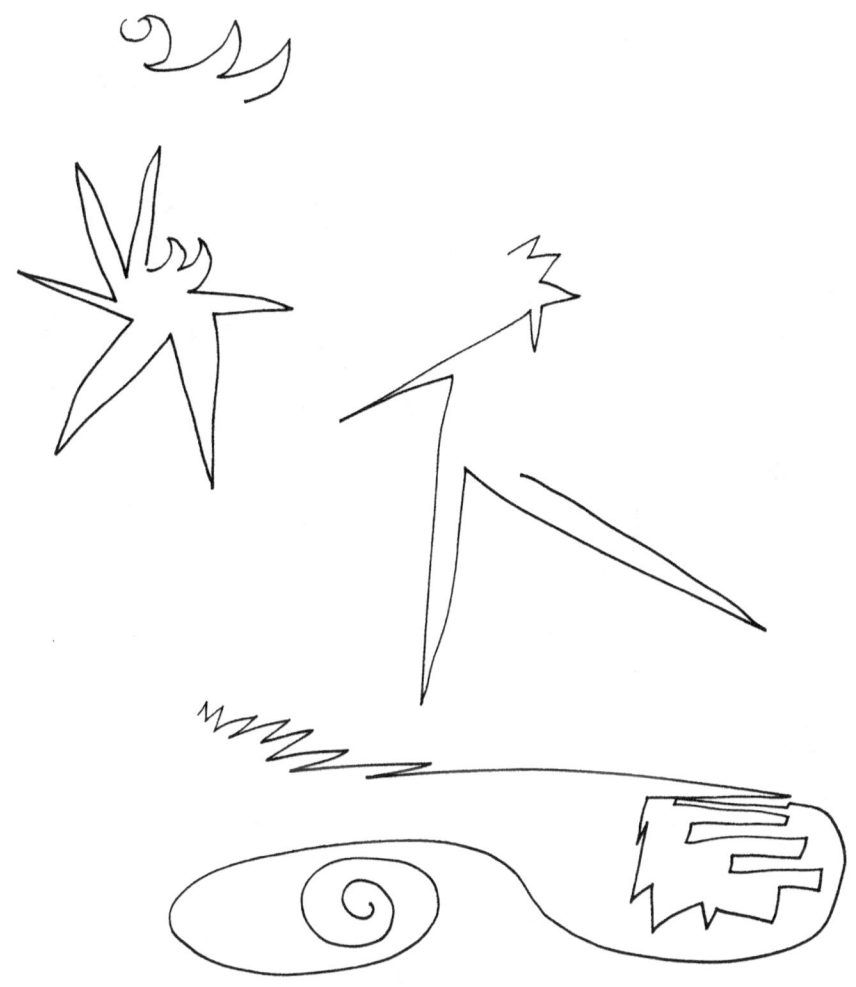

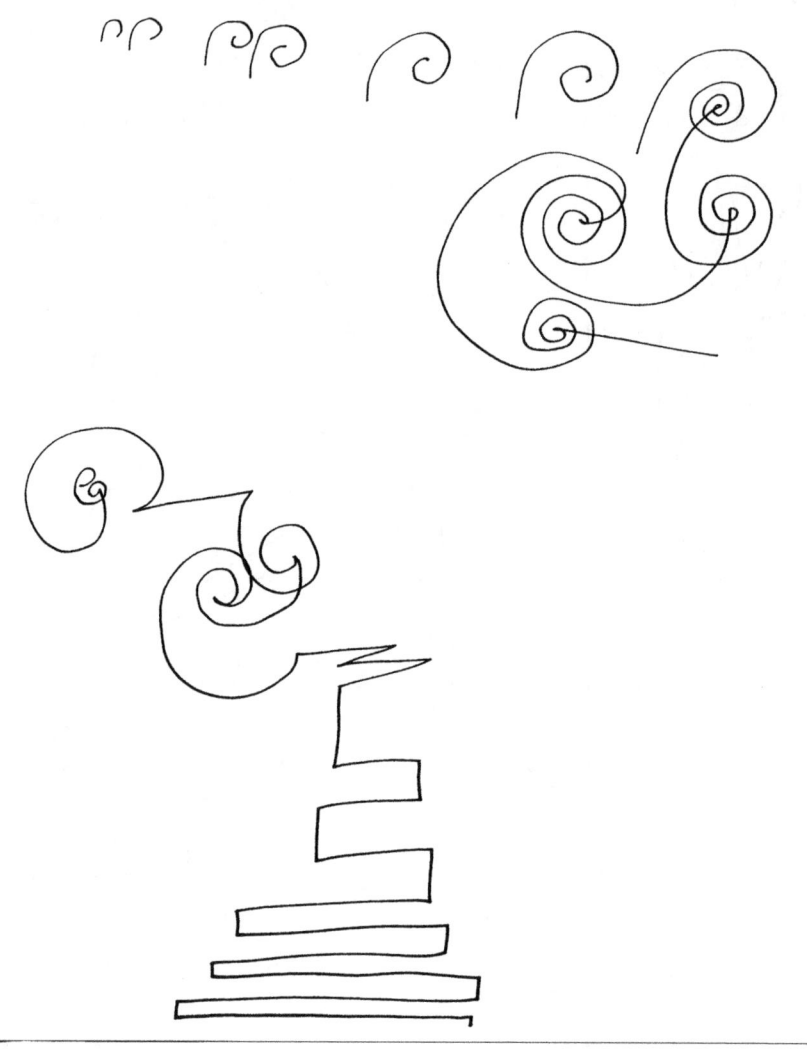

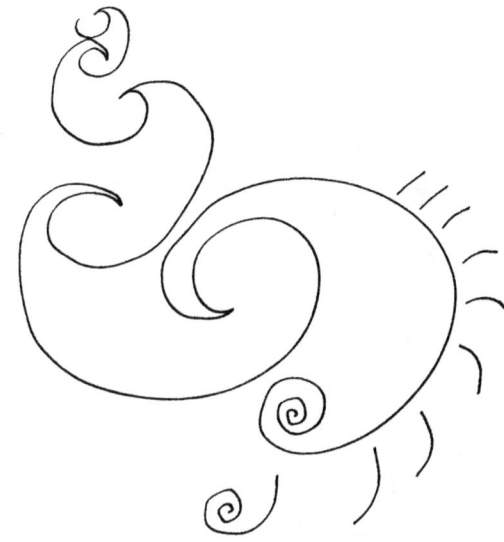

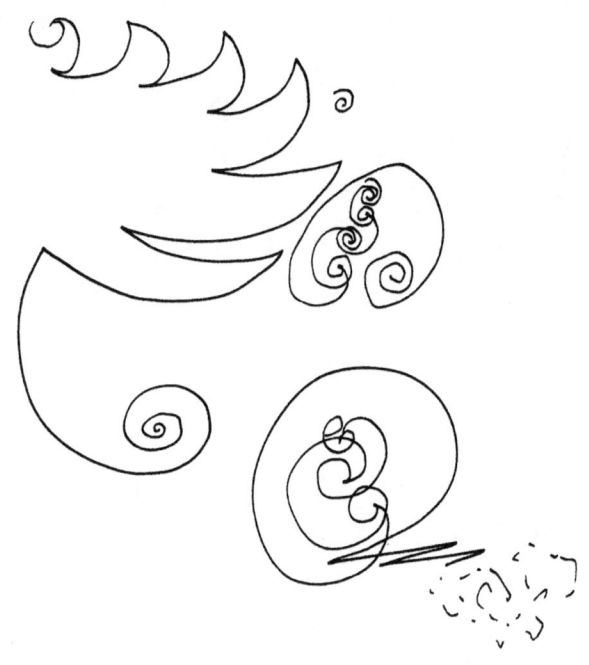

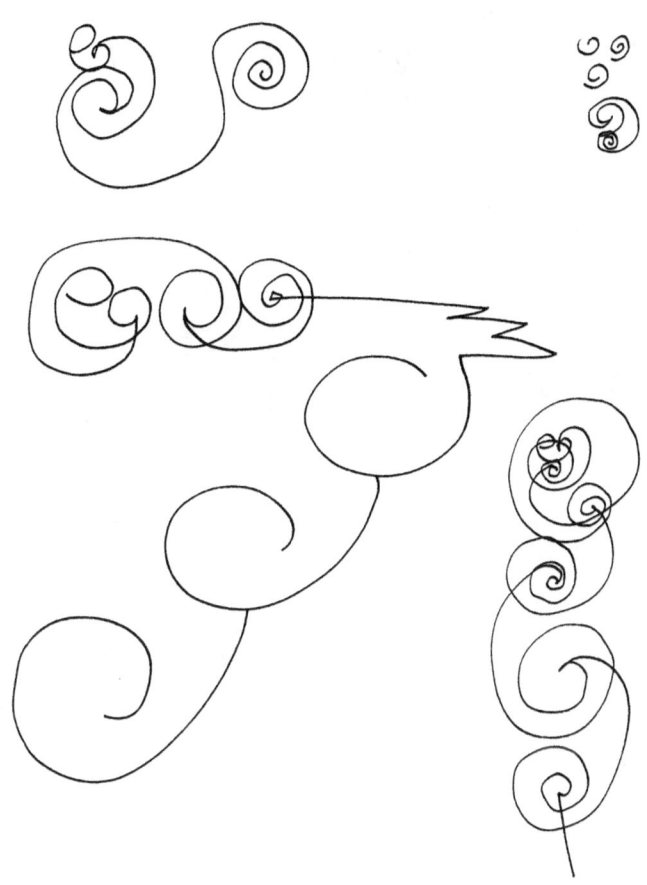

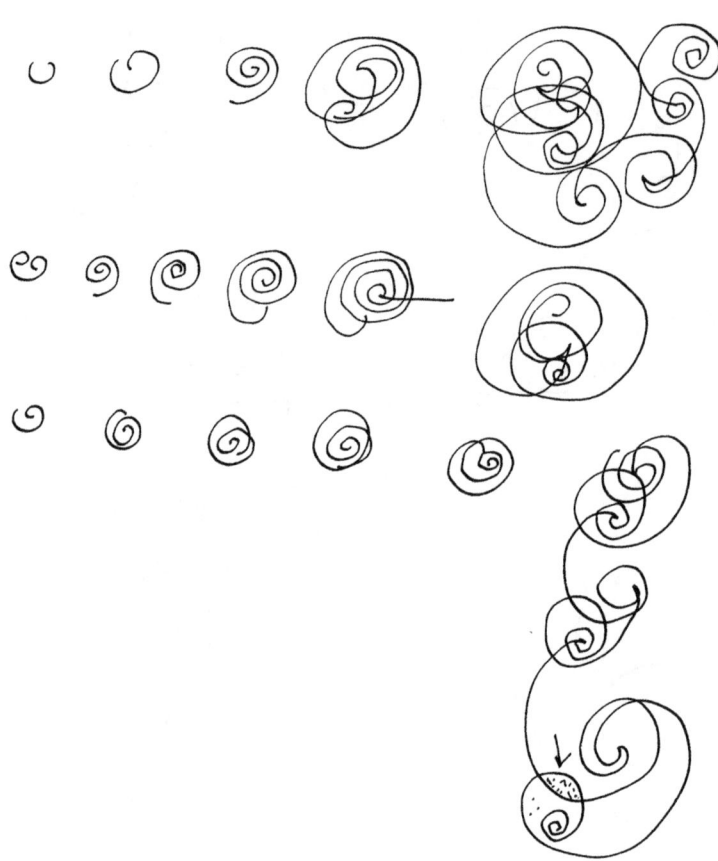

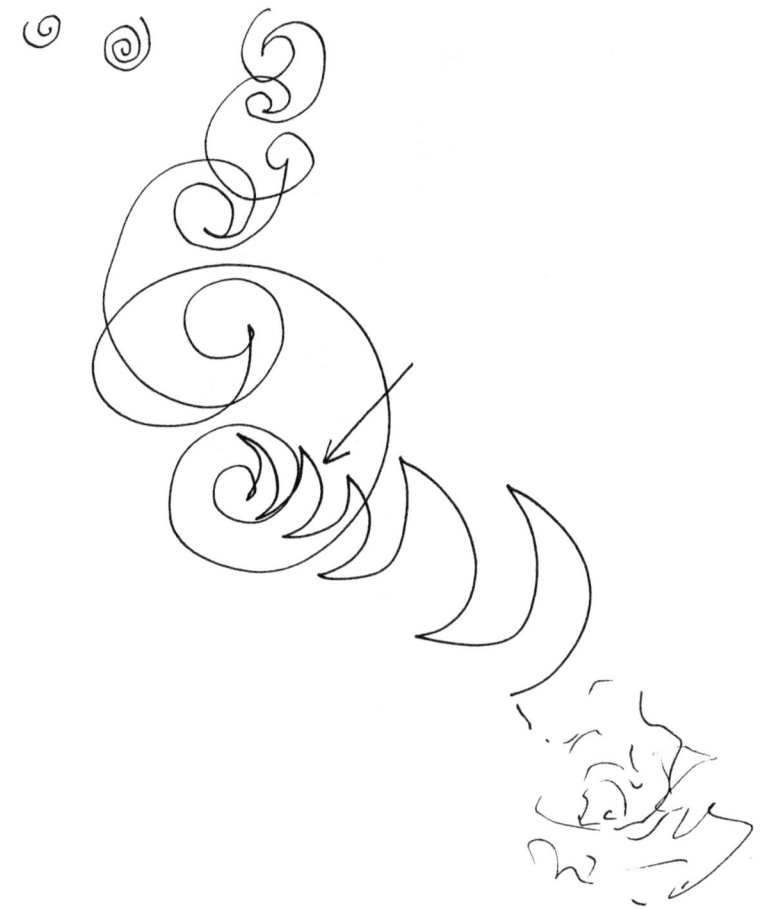

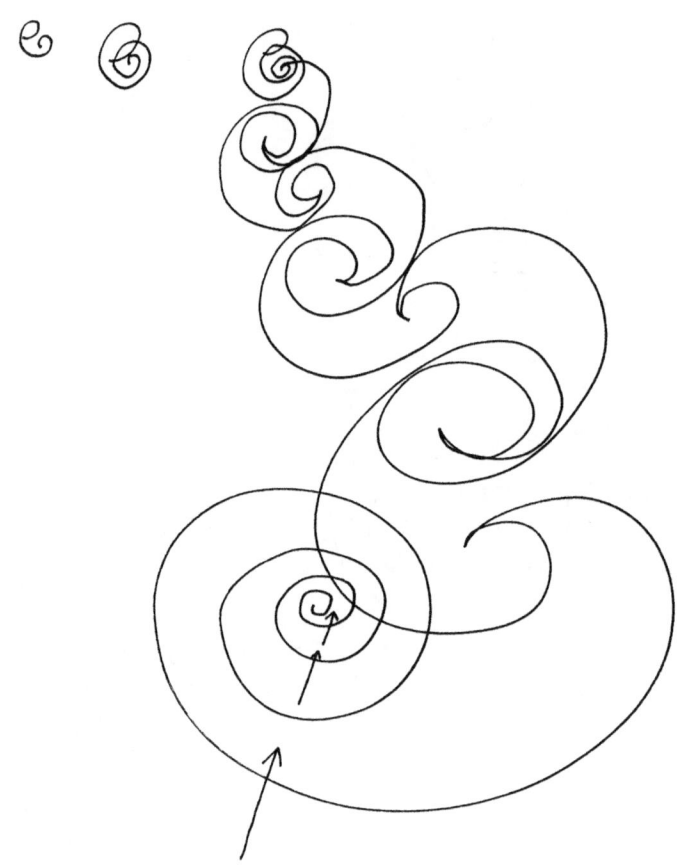

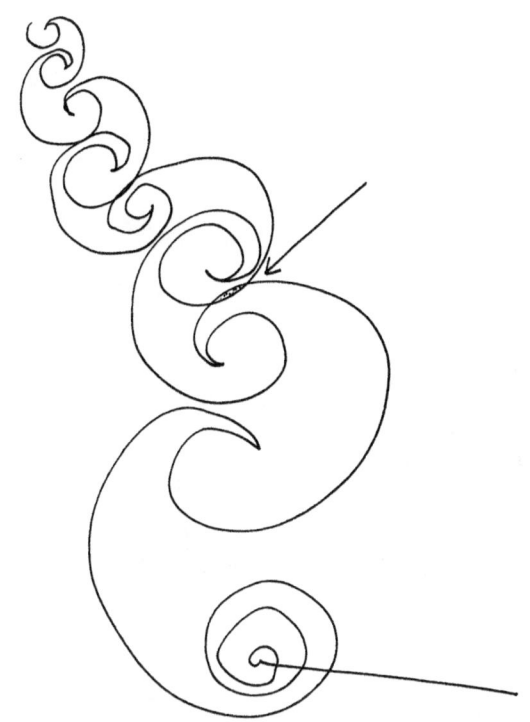

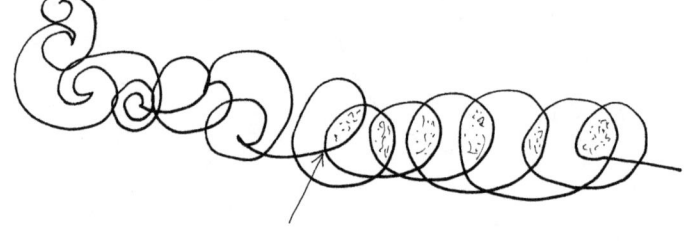

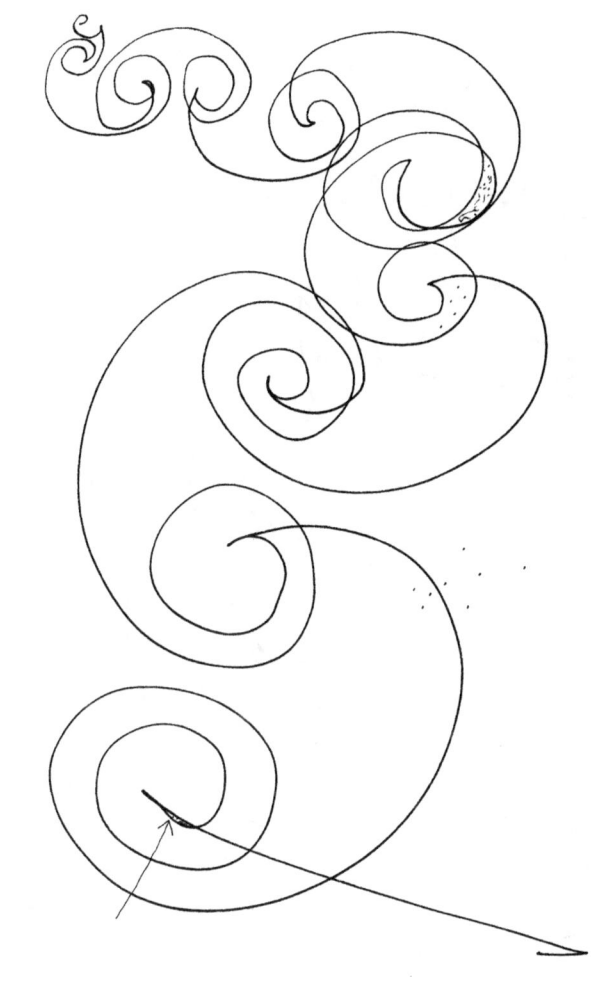

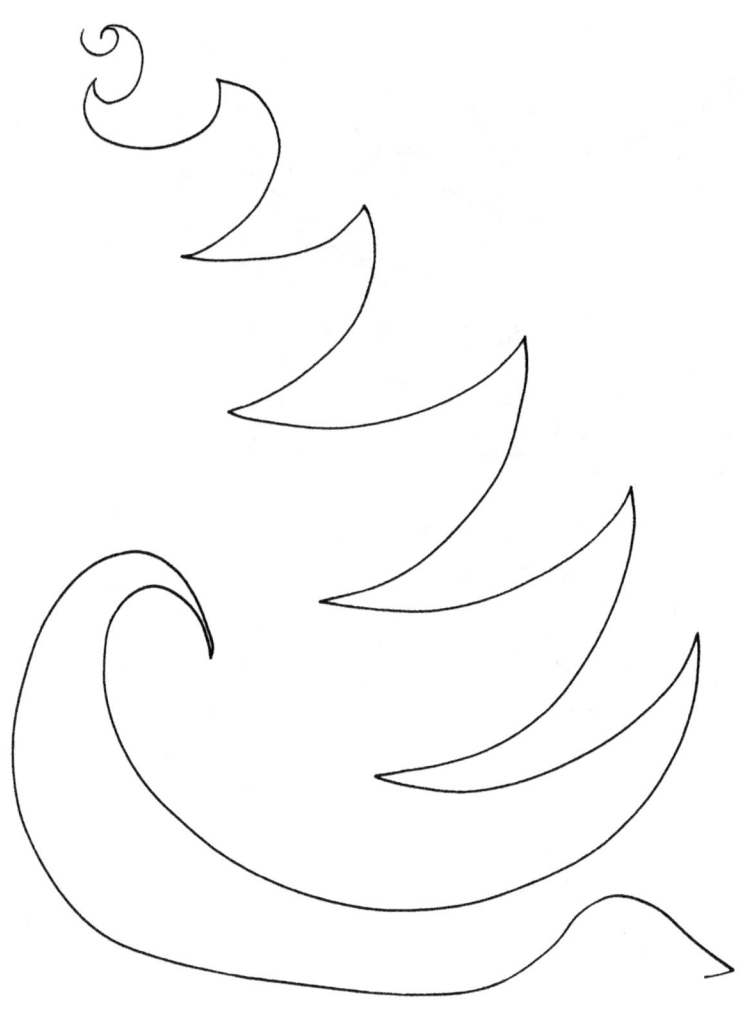

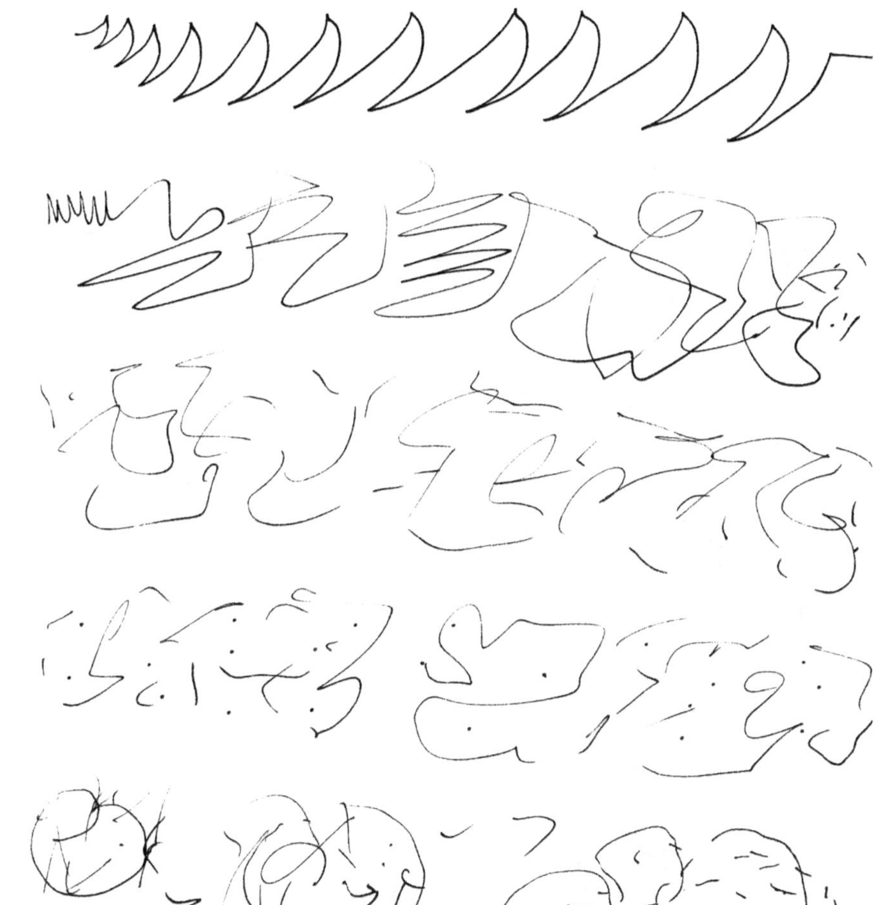

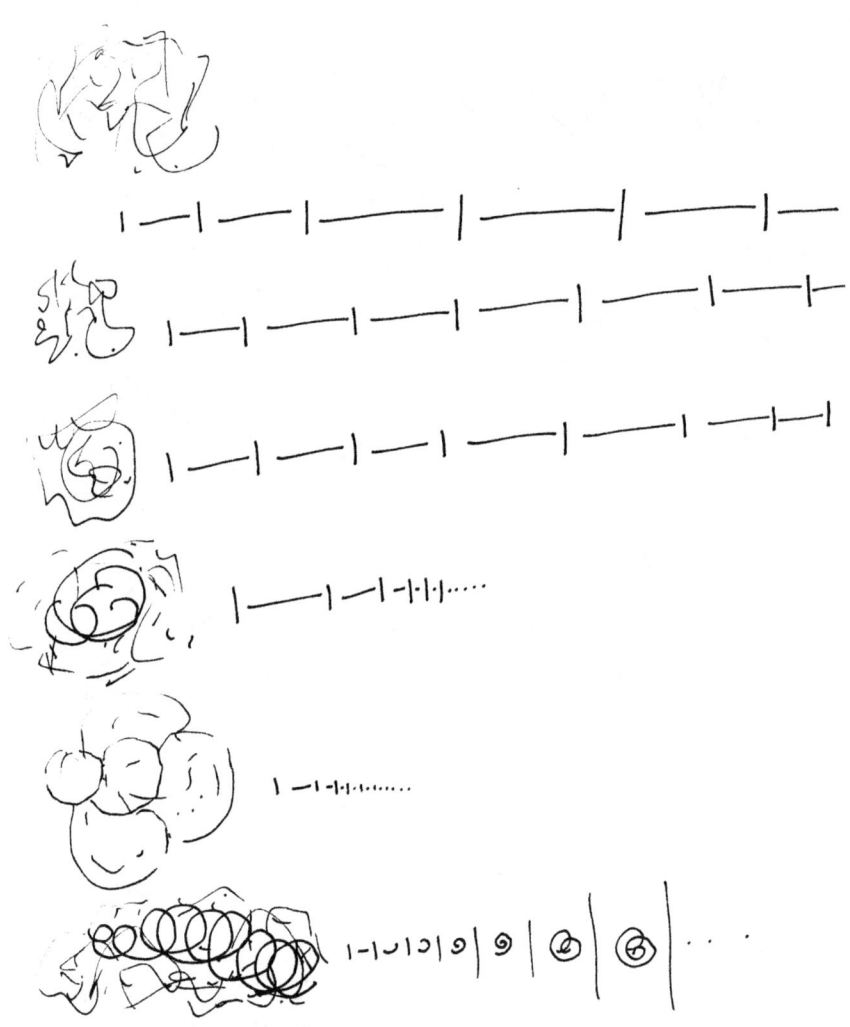

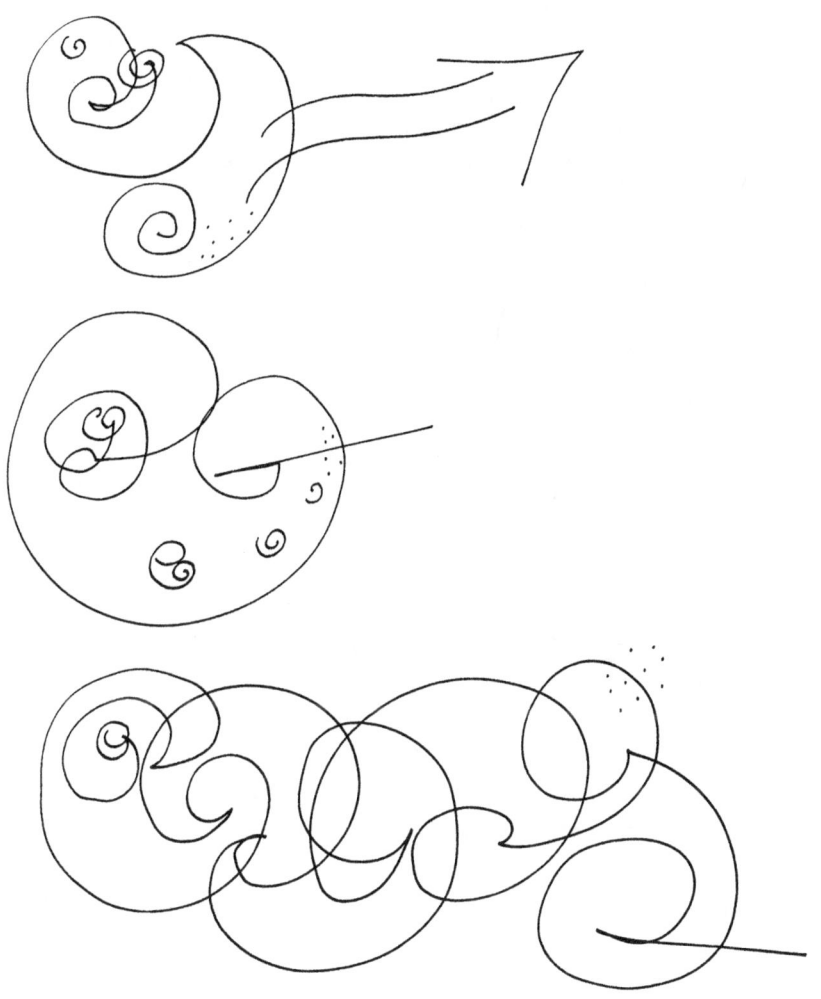

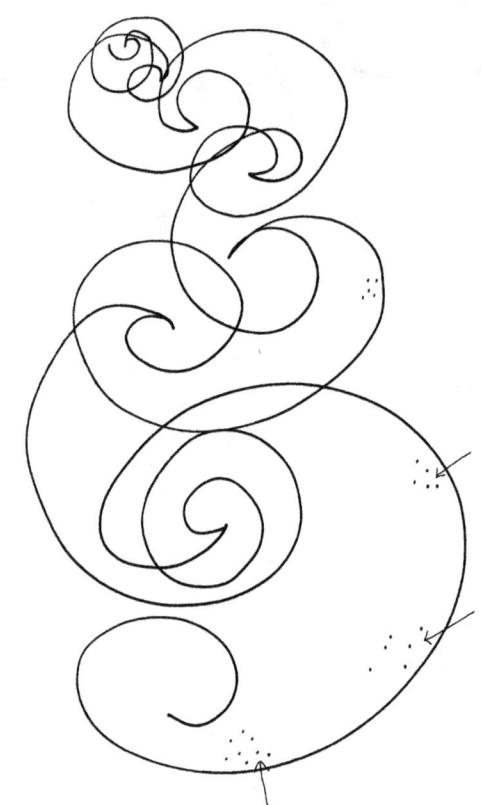

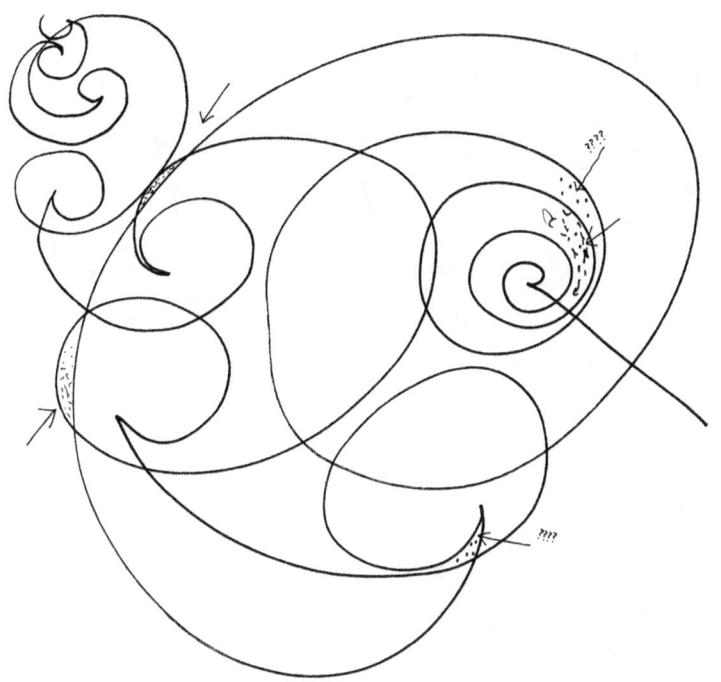

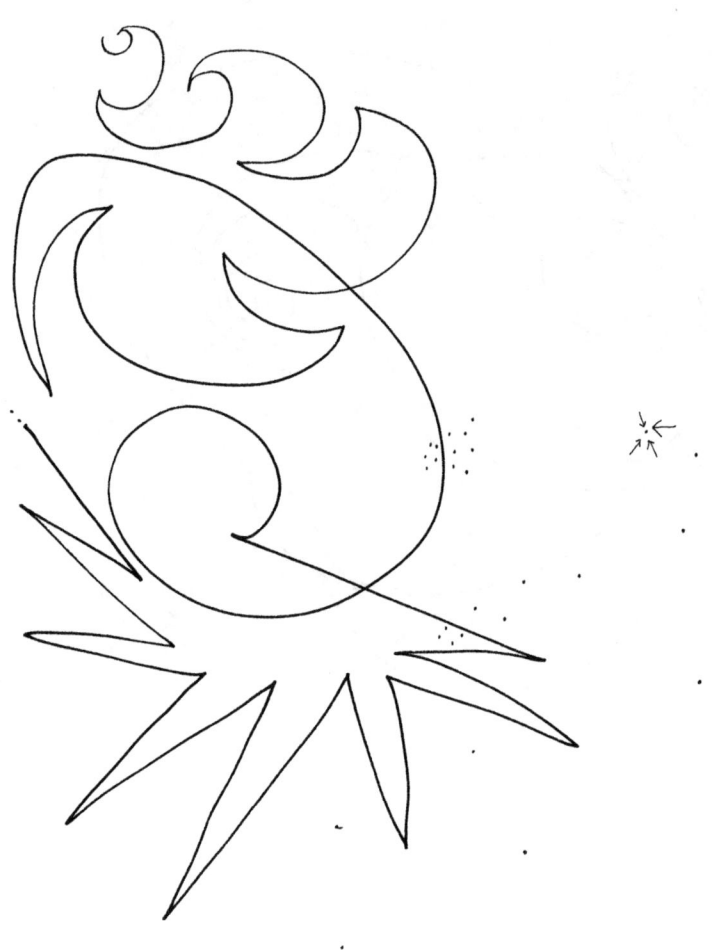

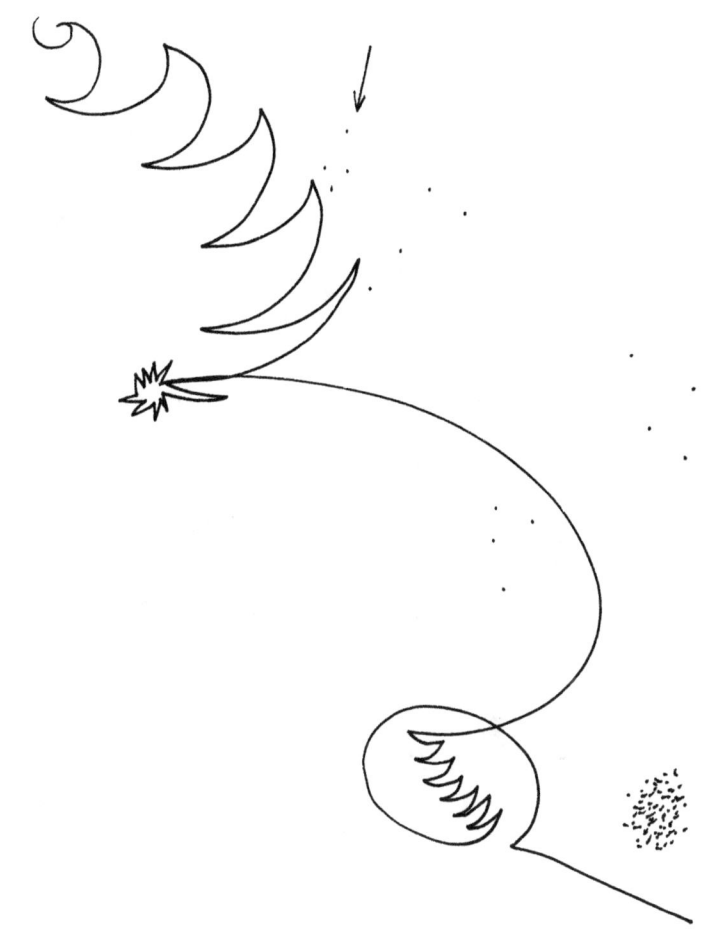

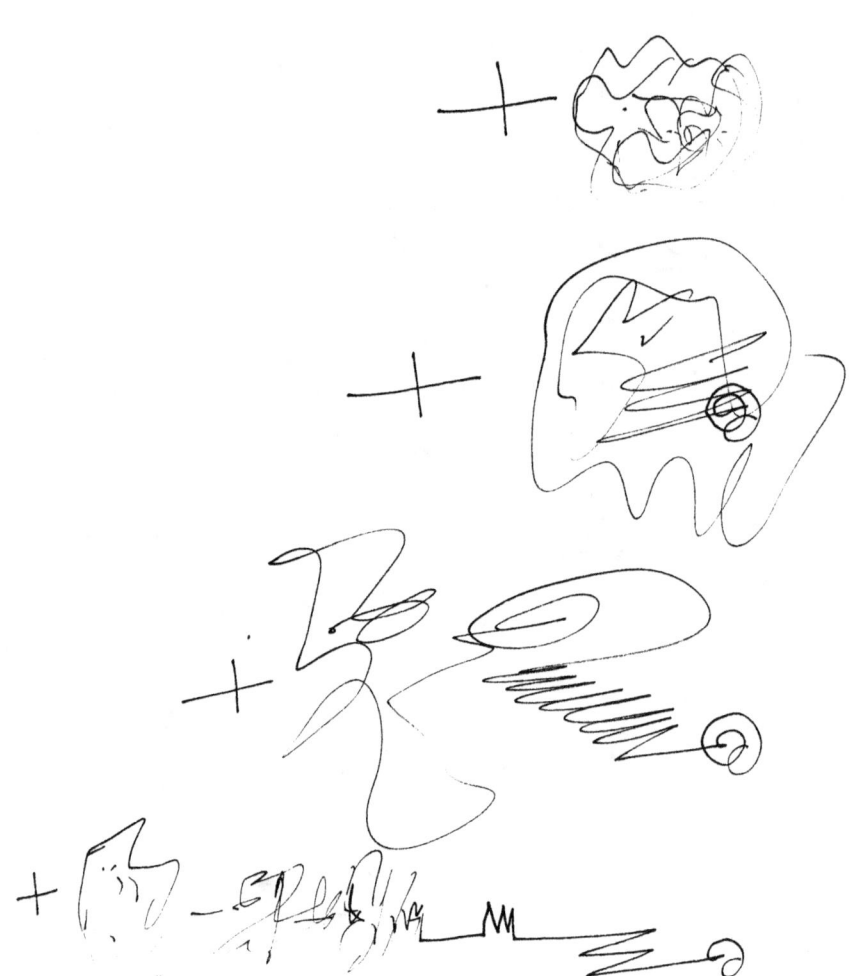

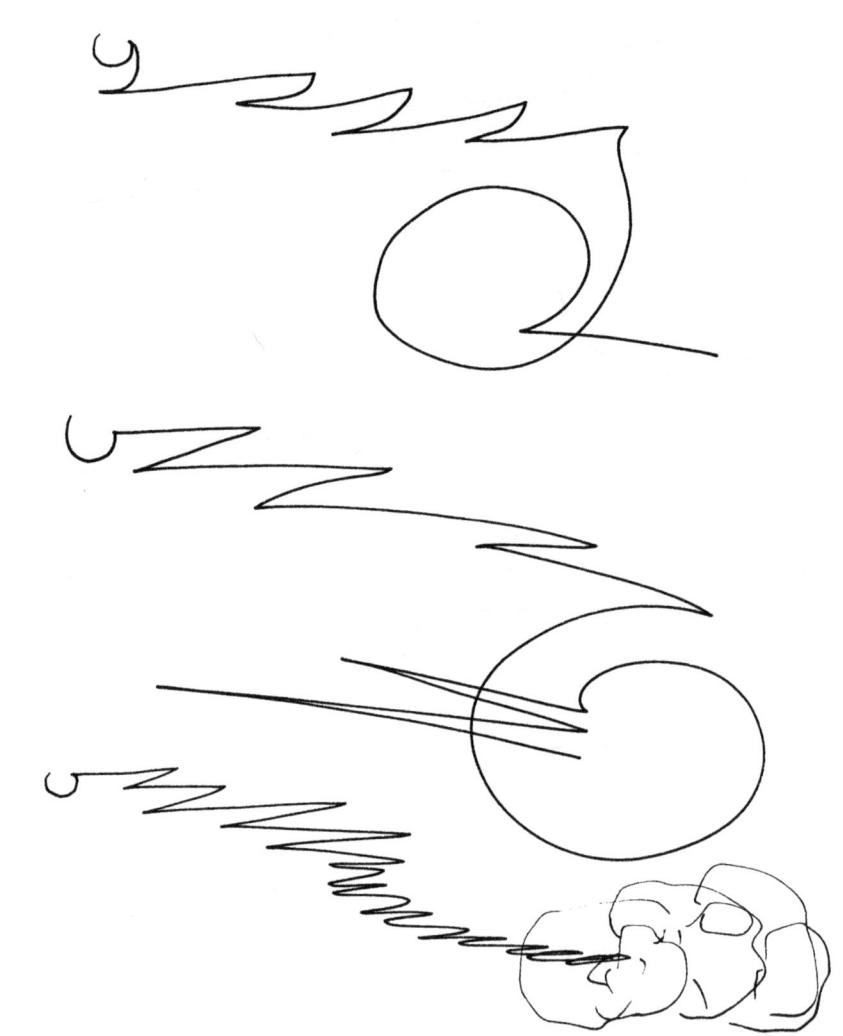

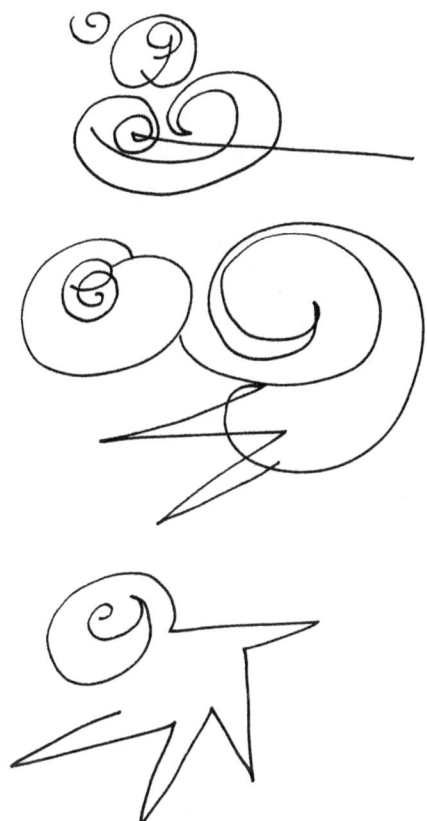

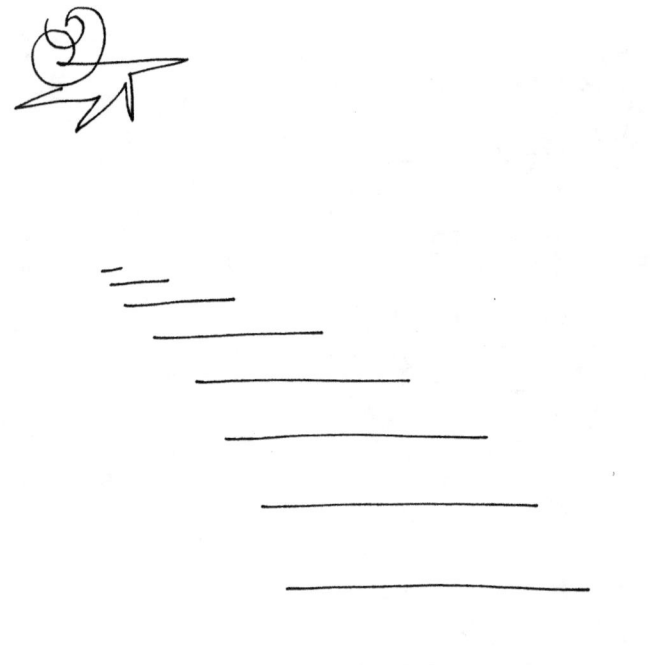

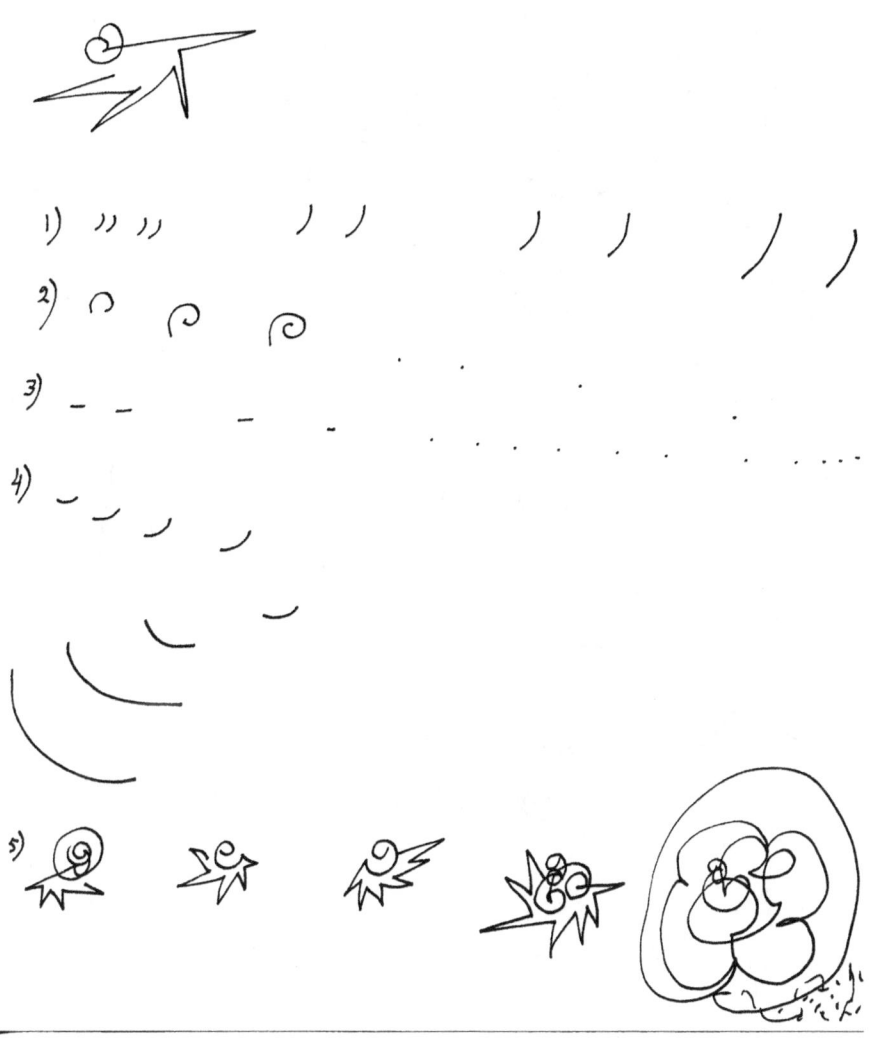

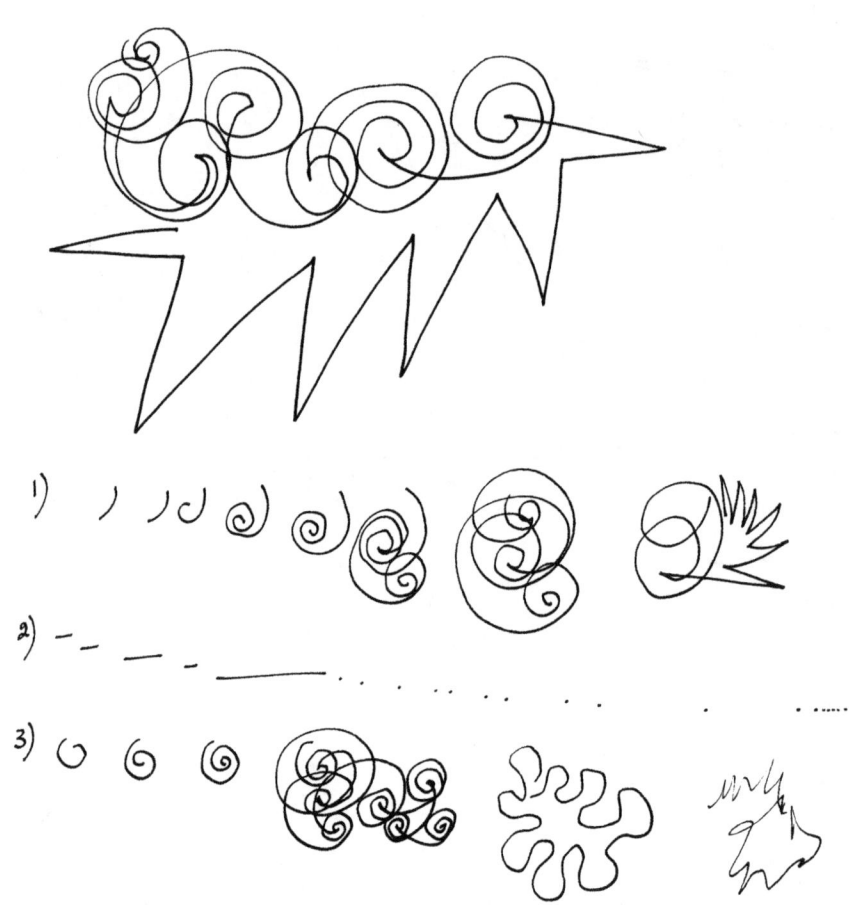

4)

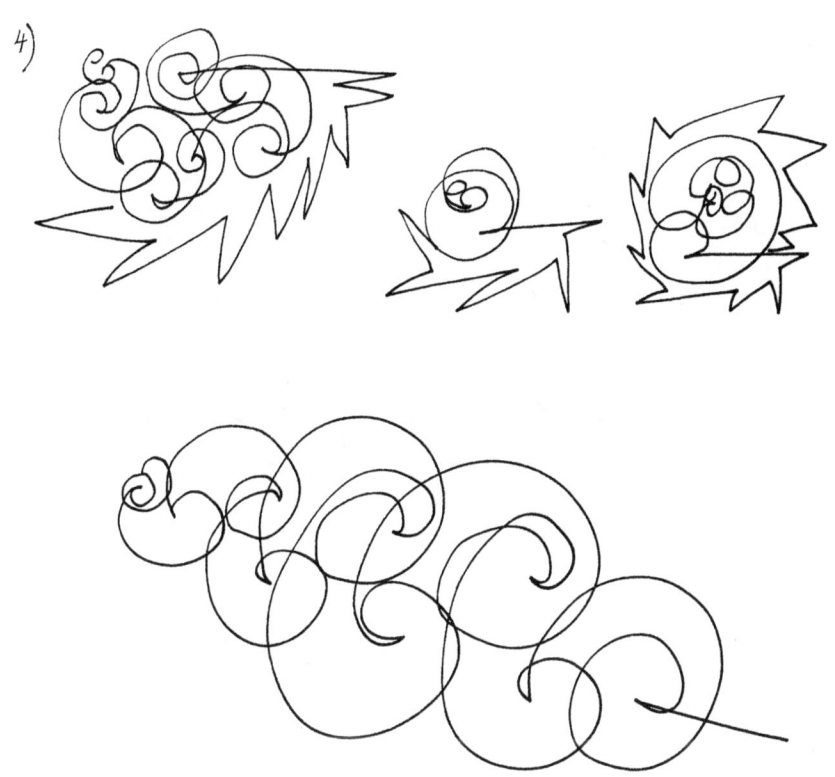

5)

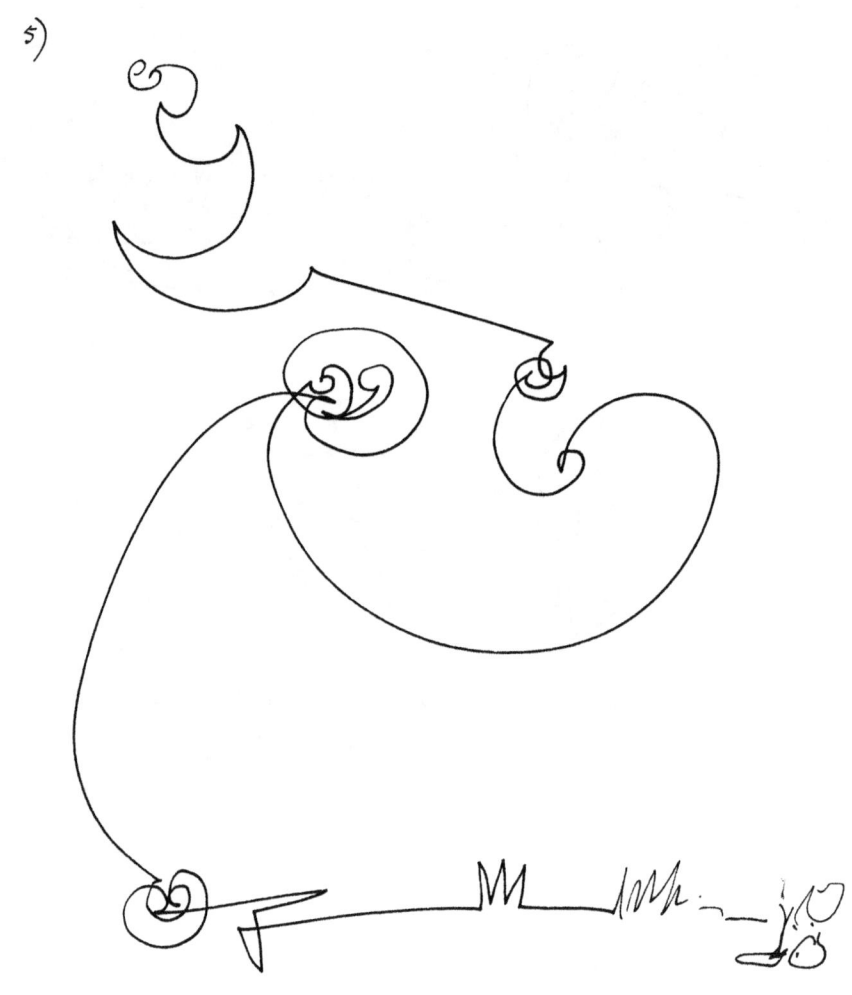

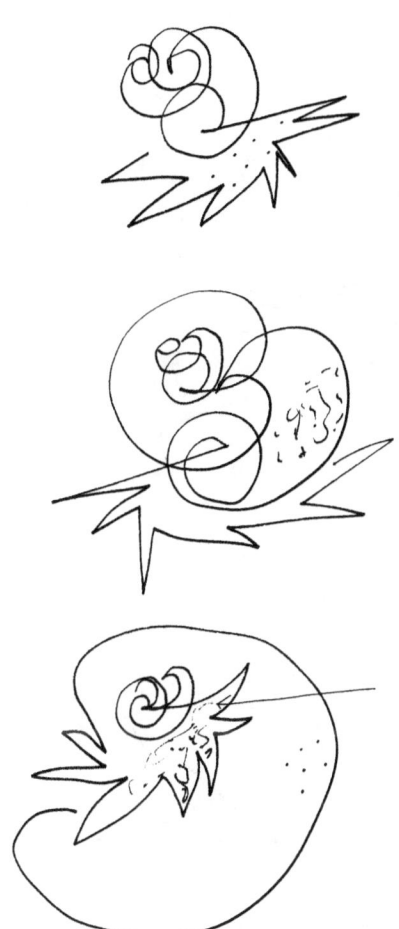

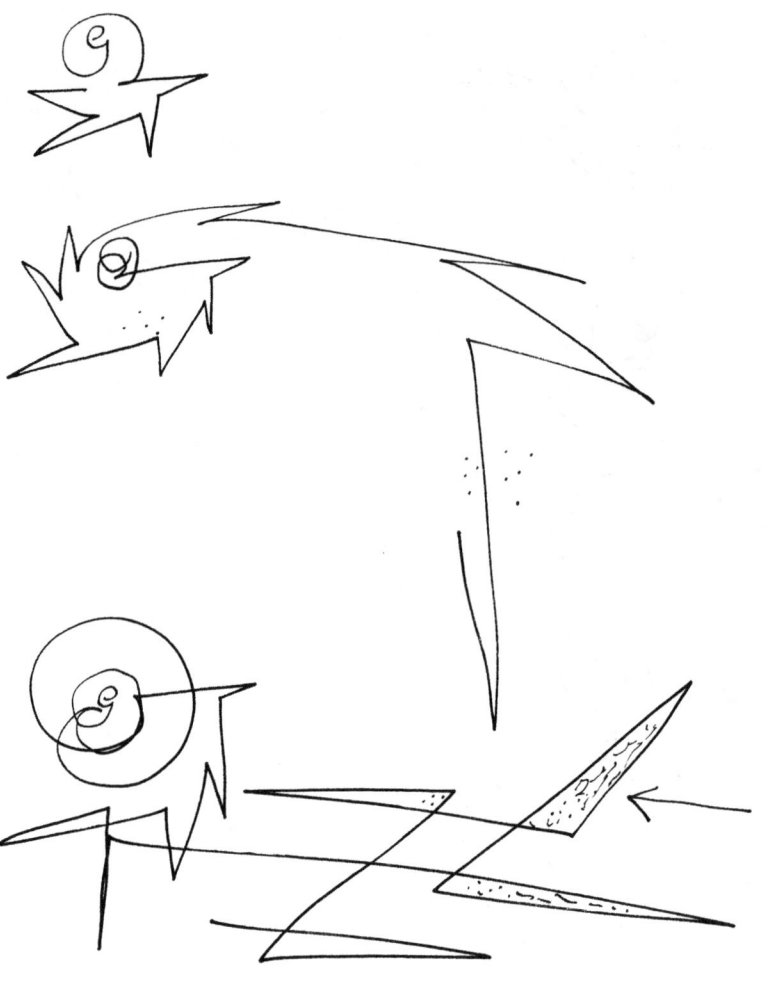

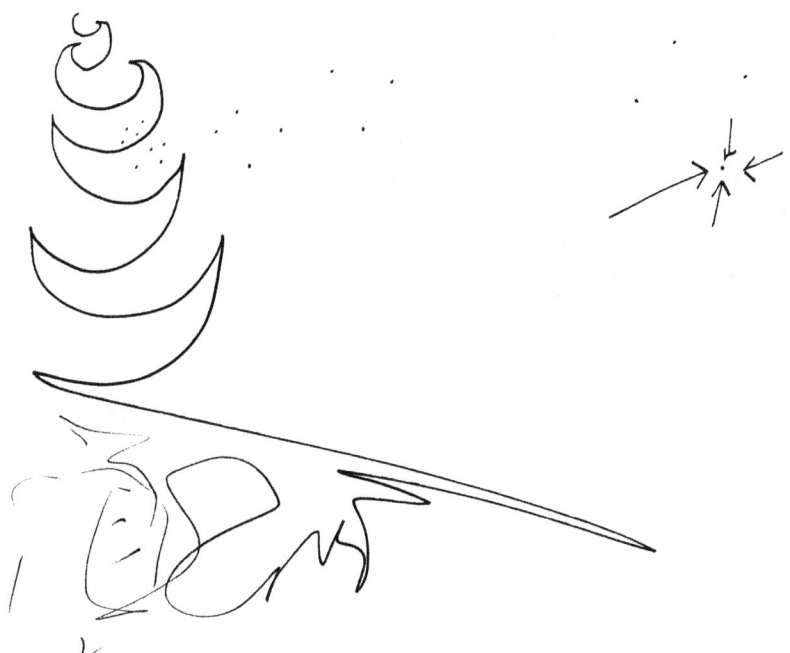

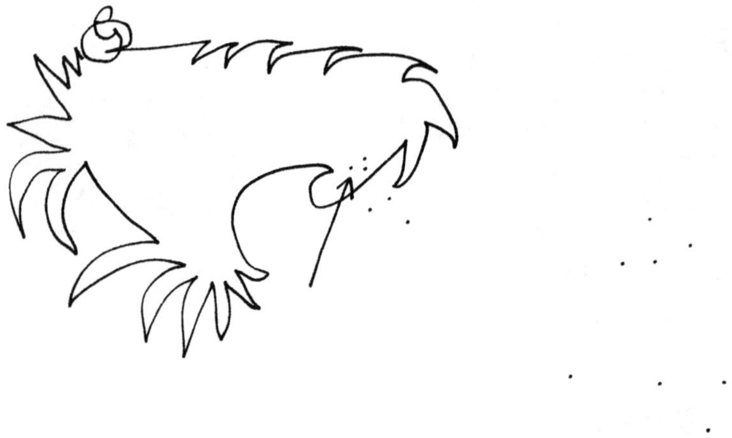

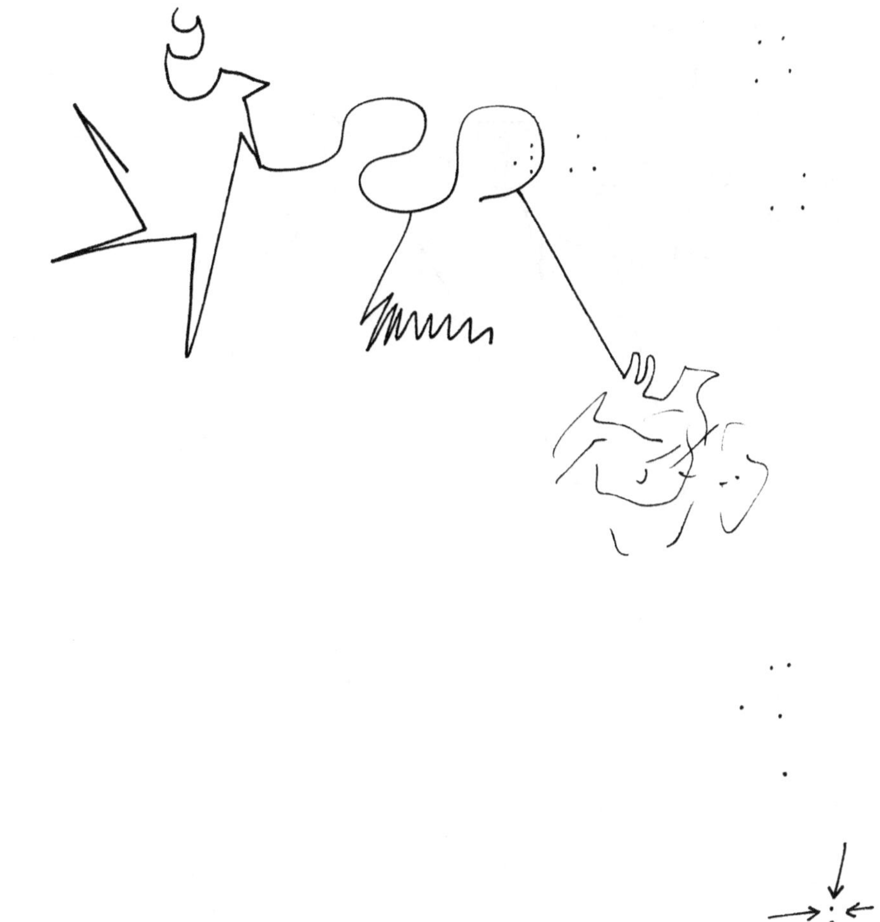

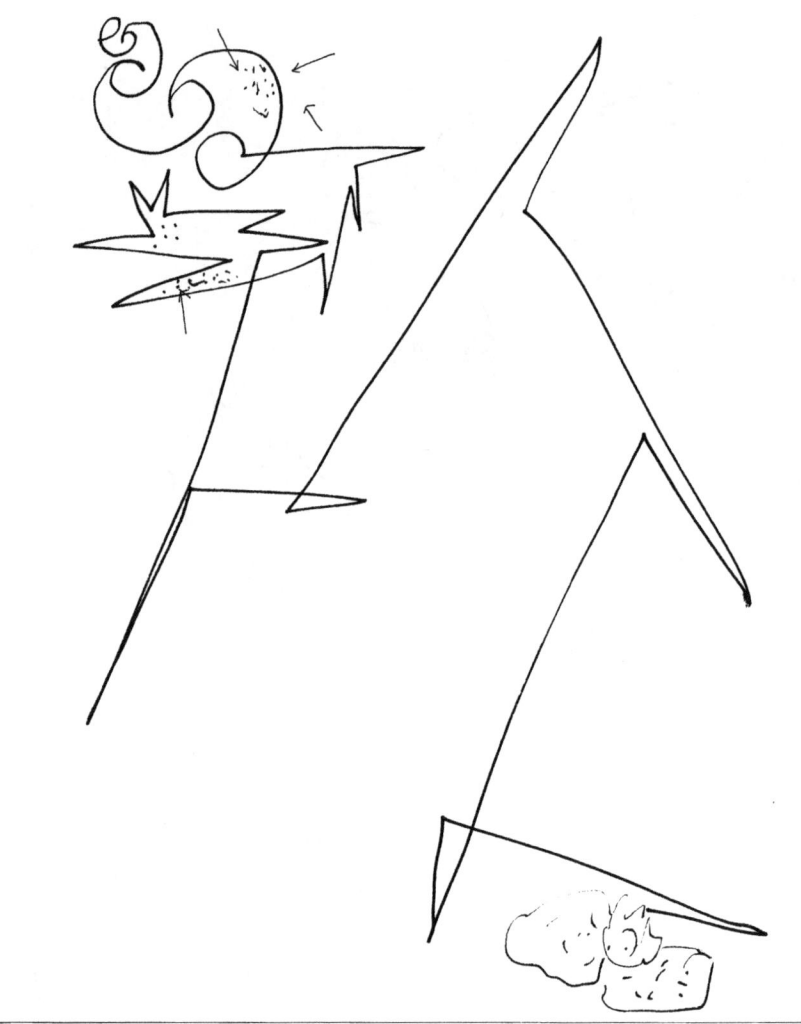

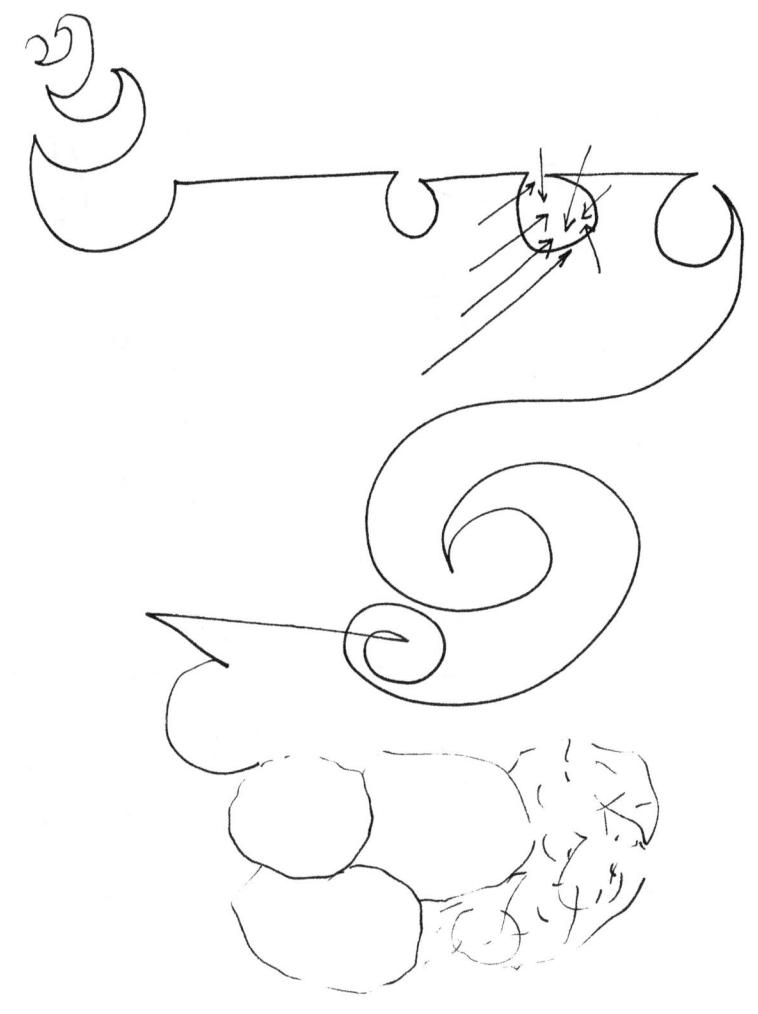

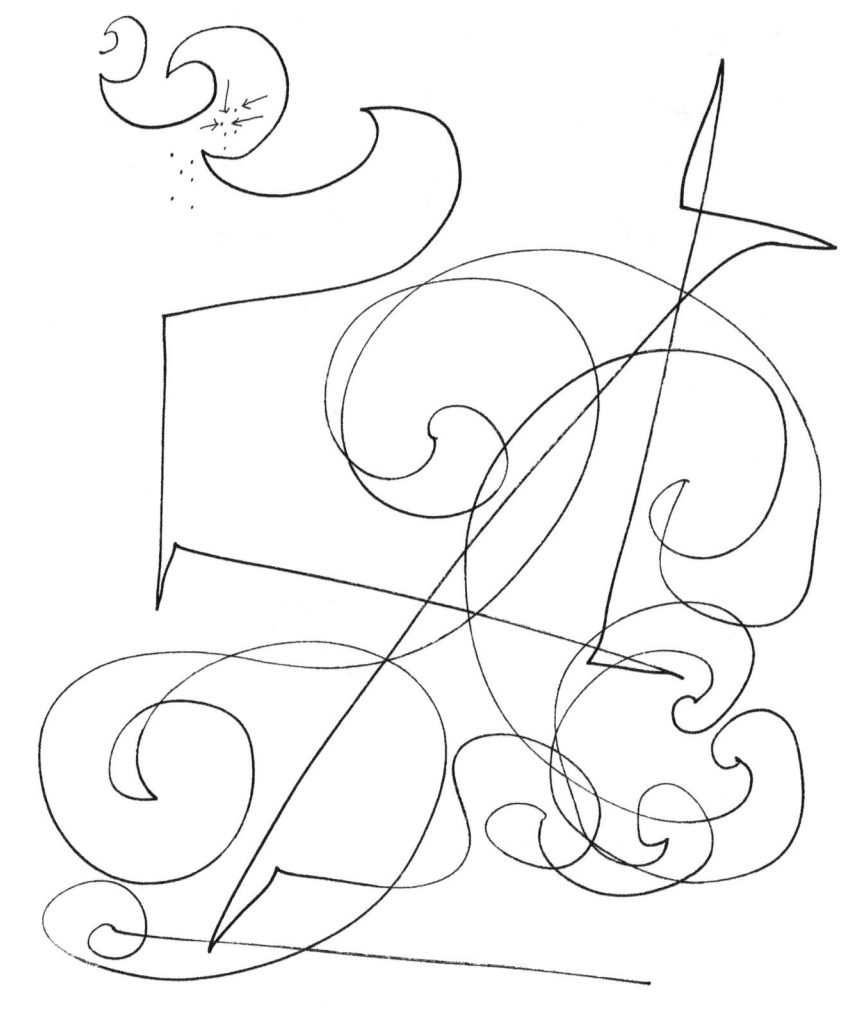

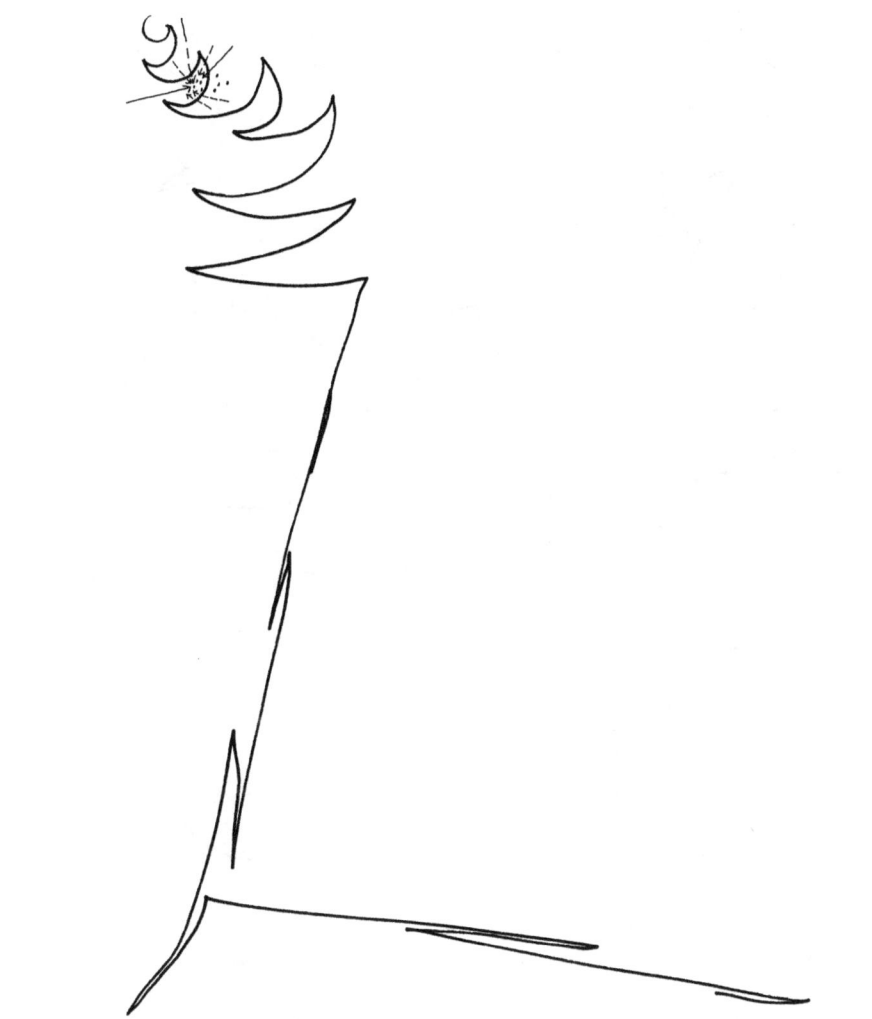

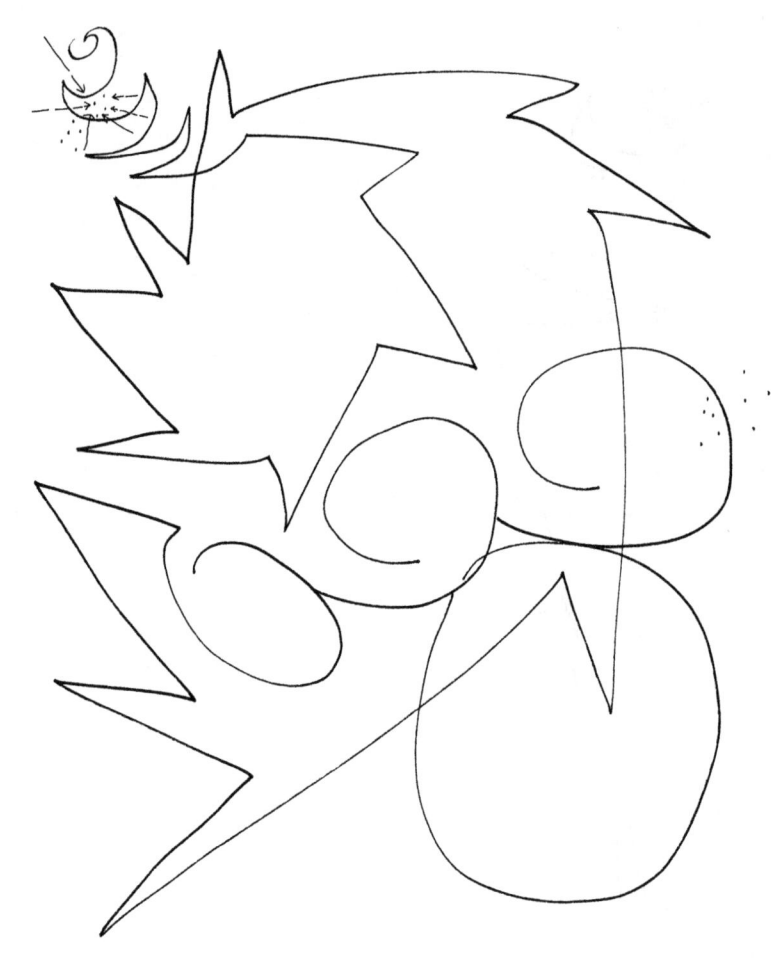

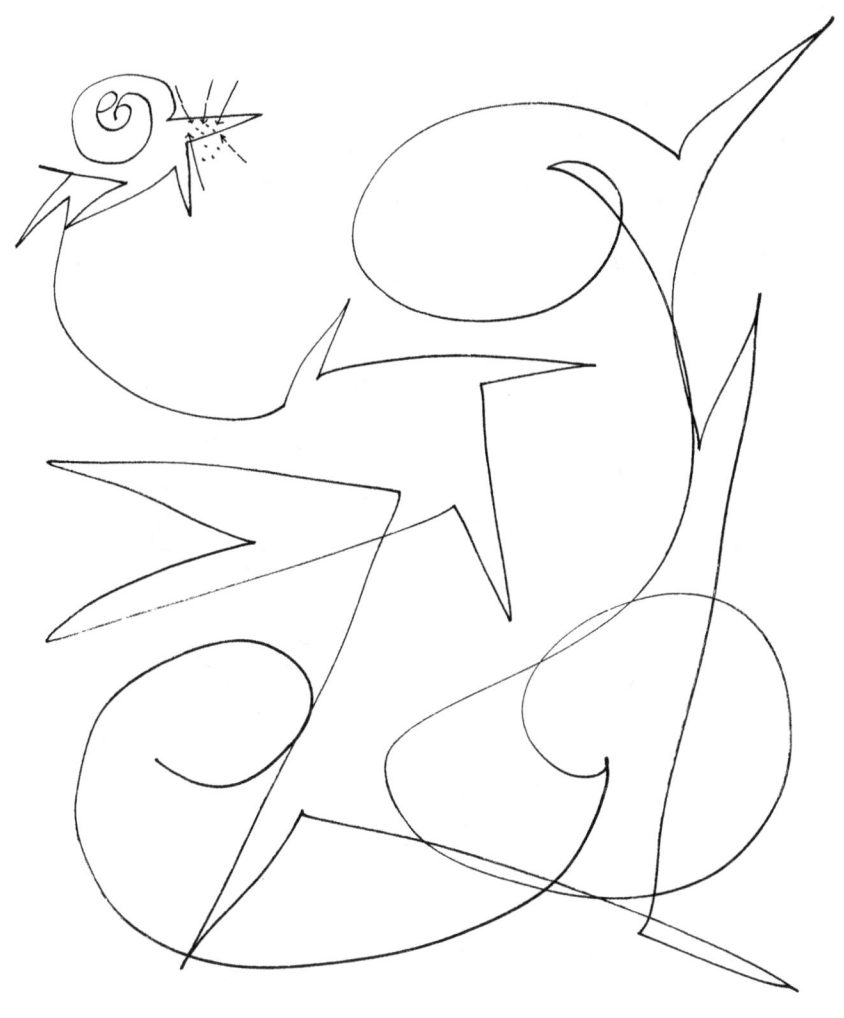

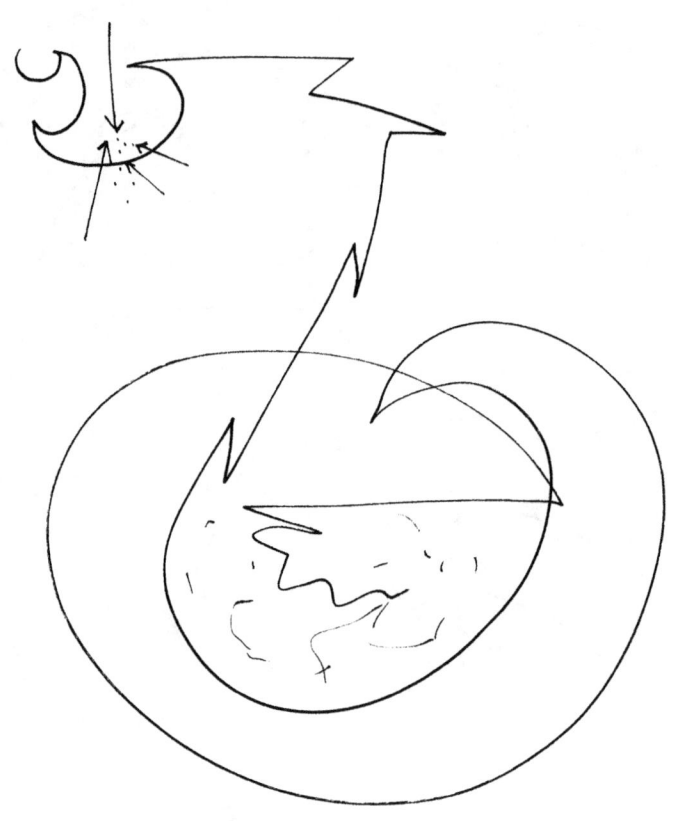

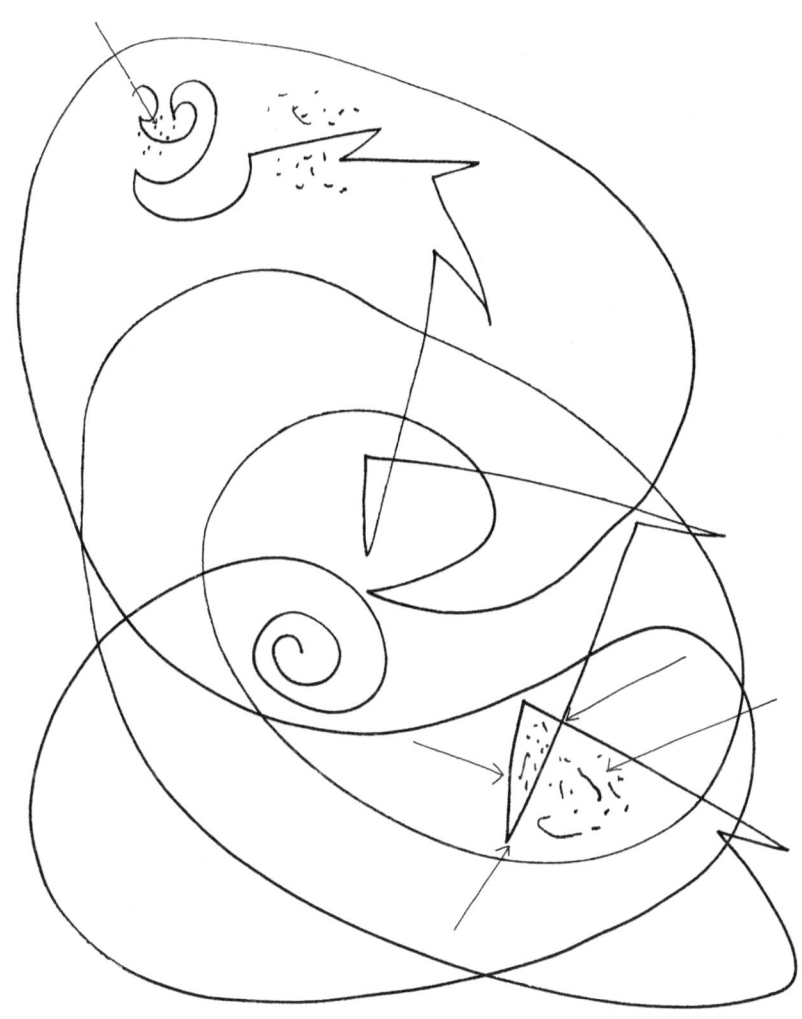

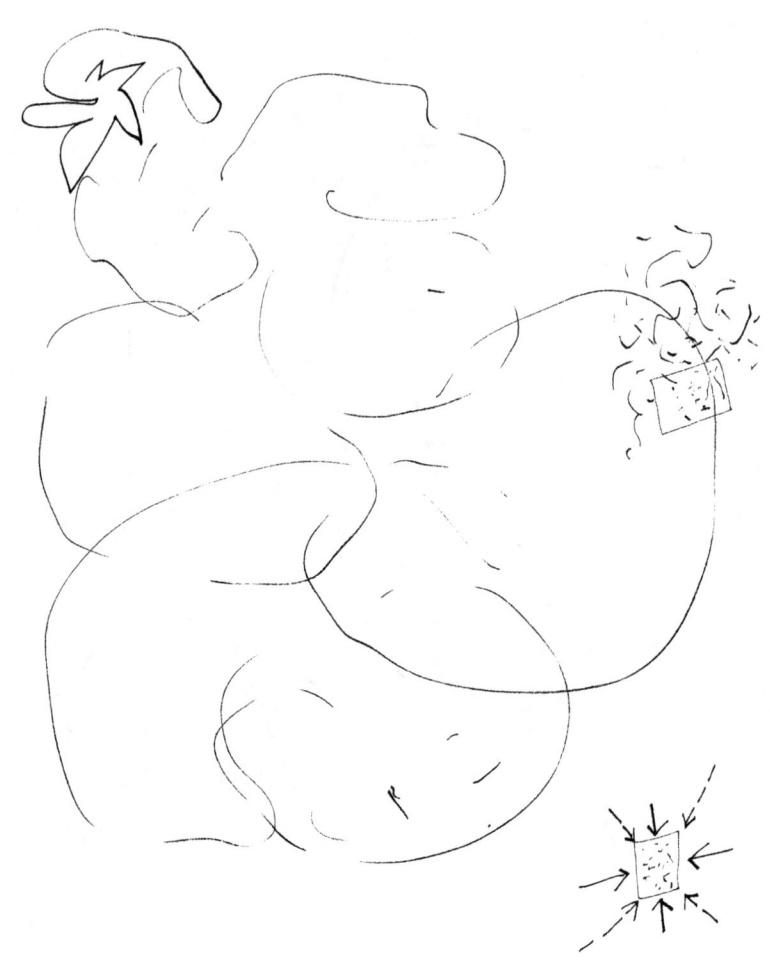

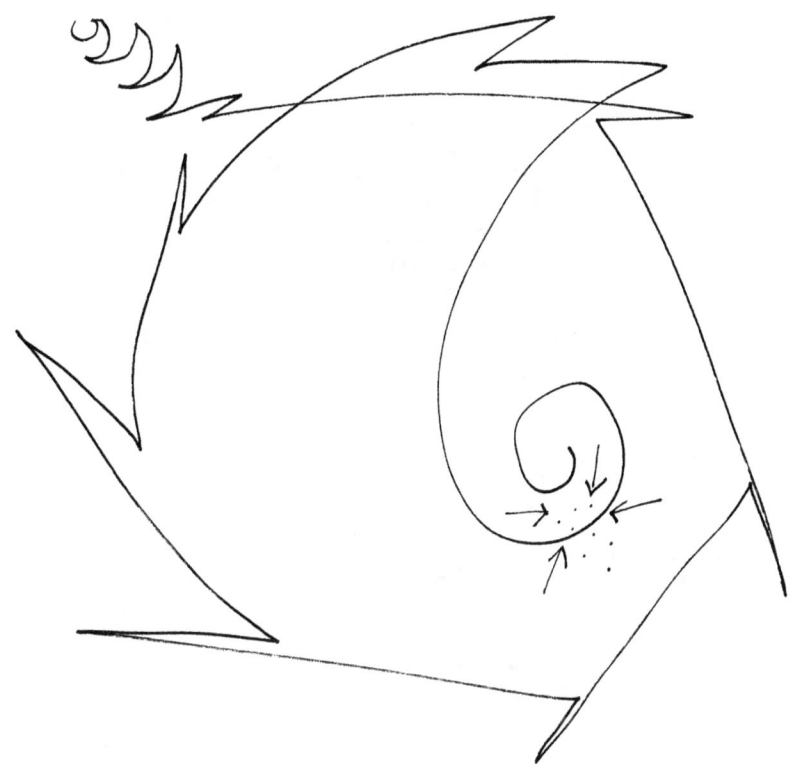

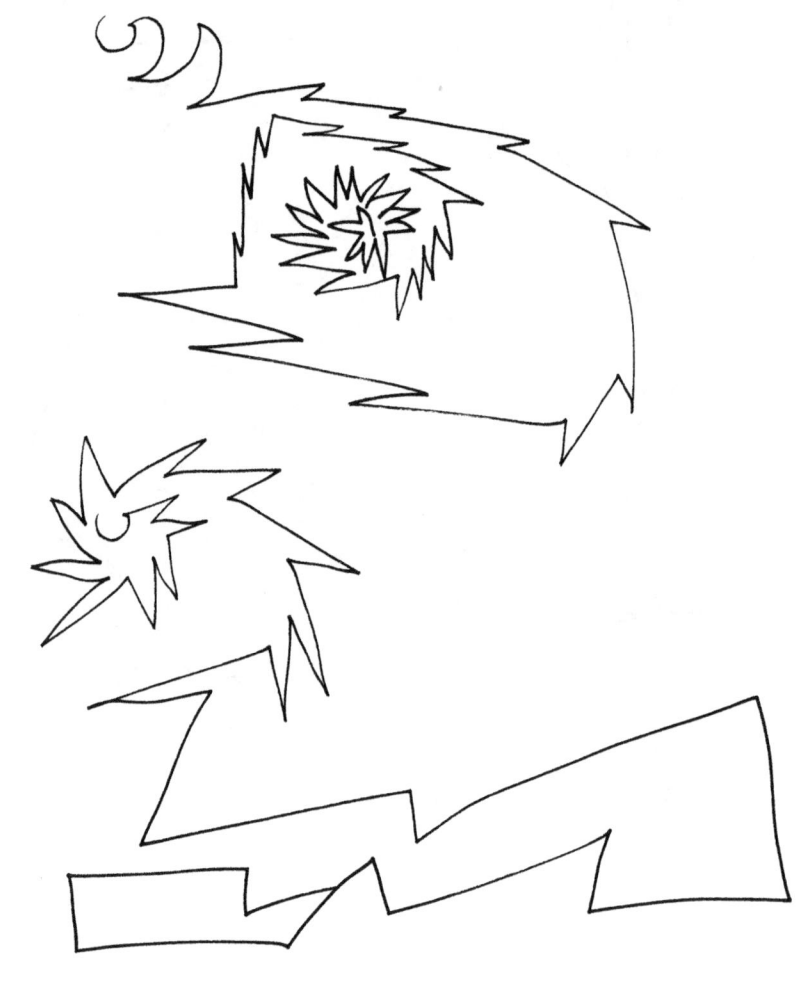

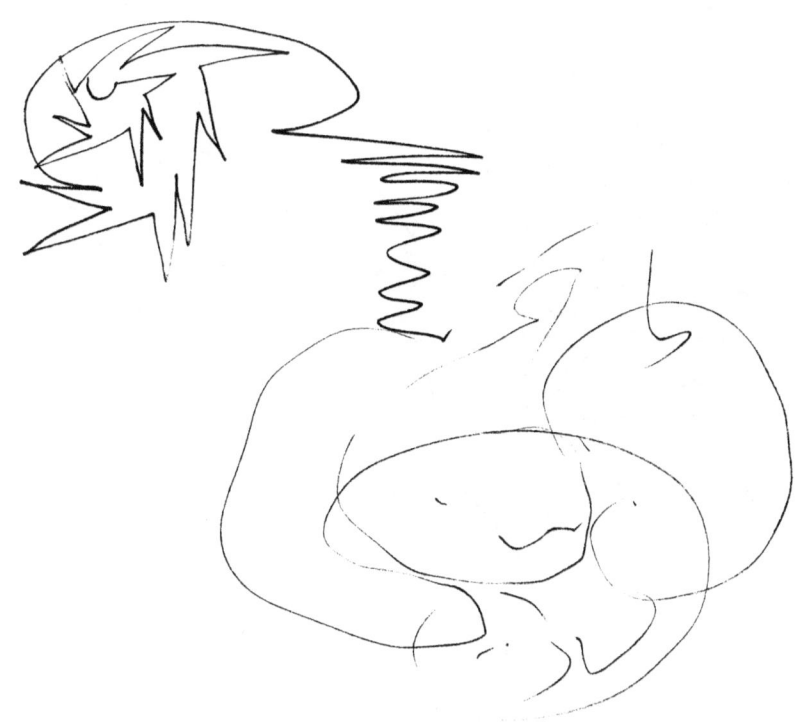

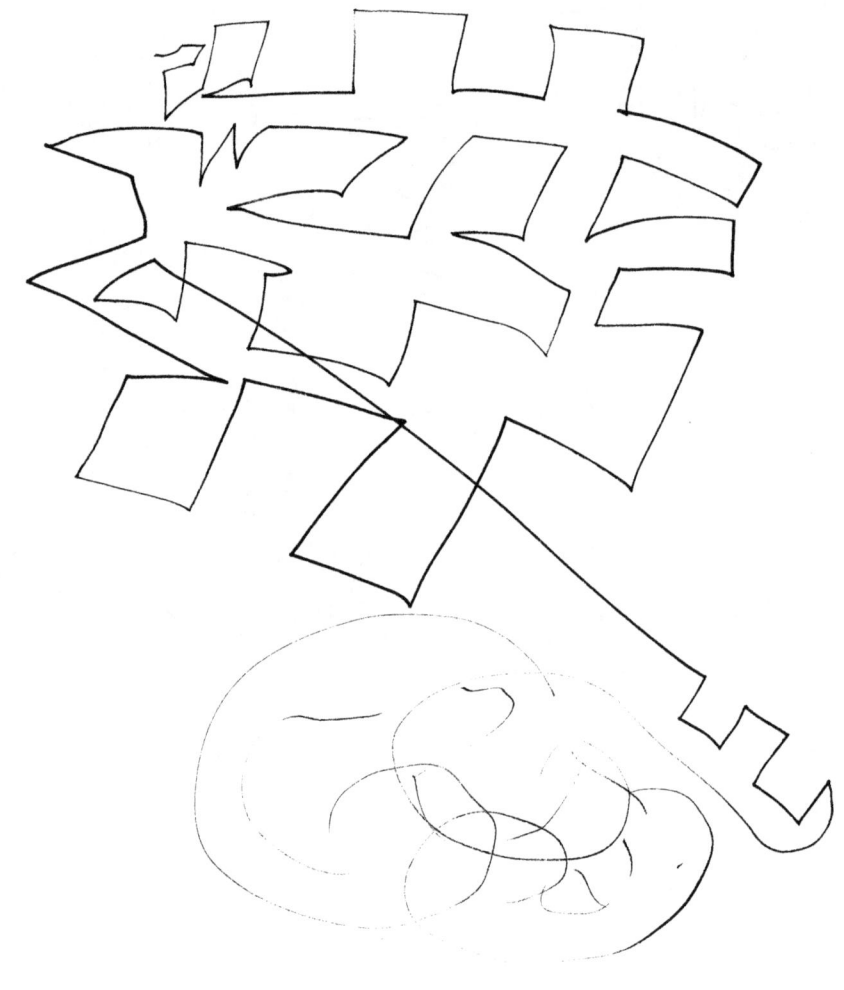

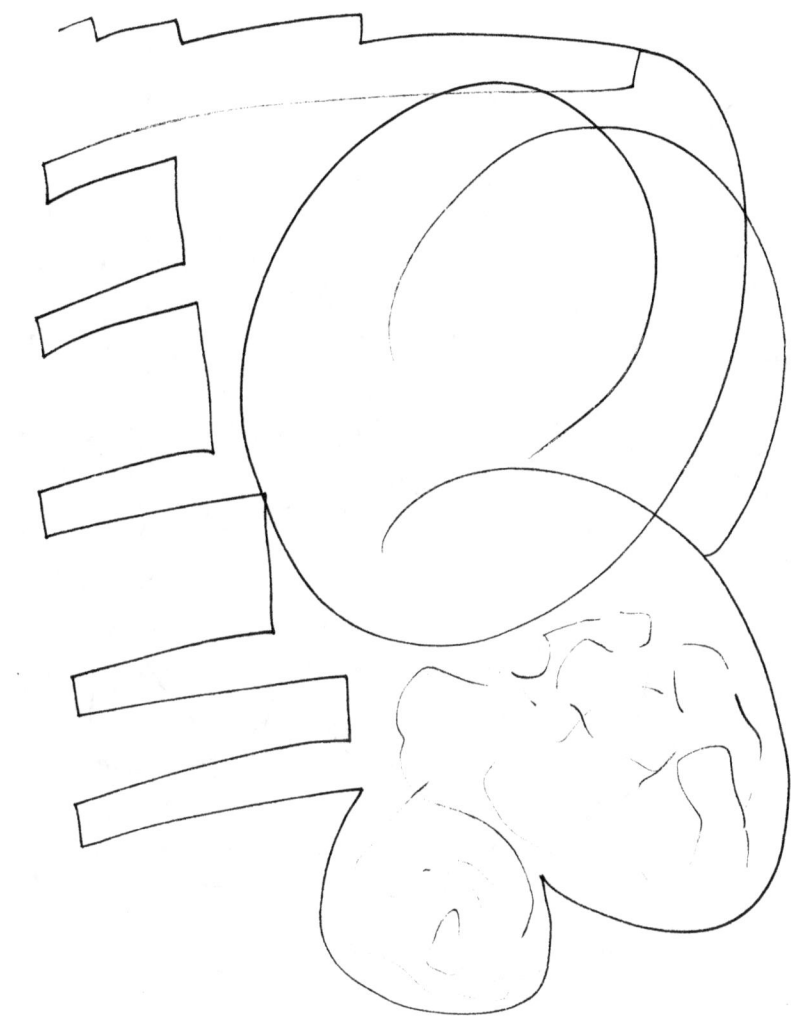

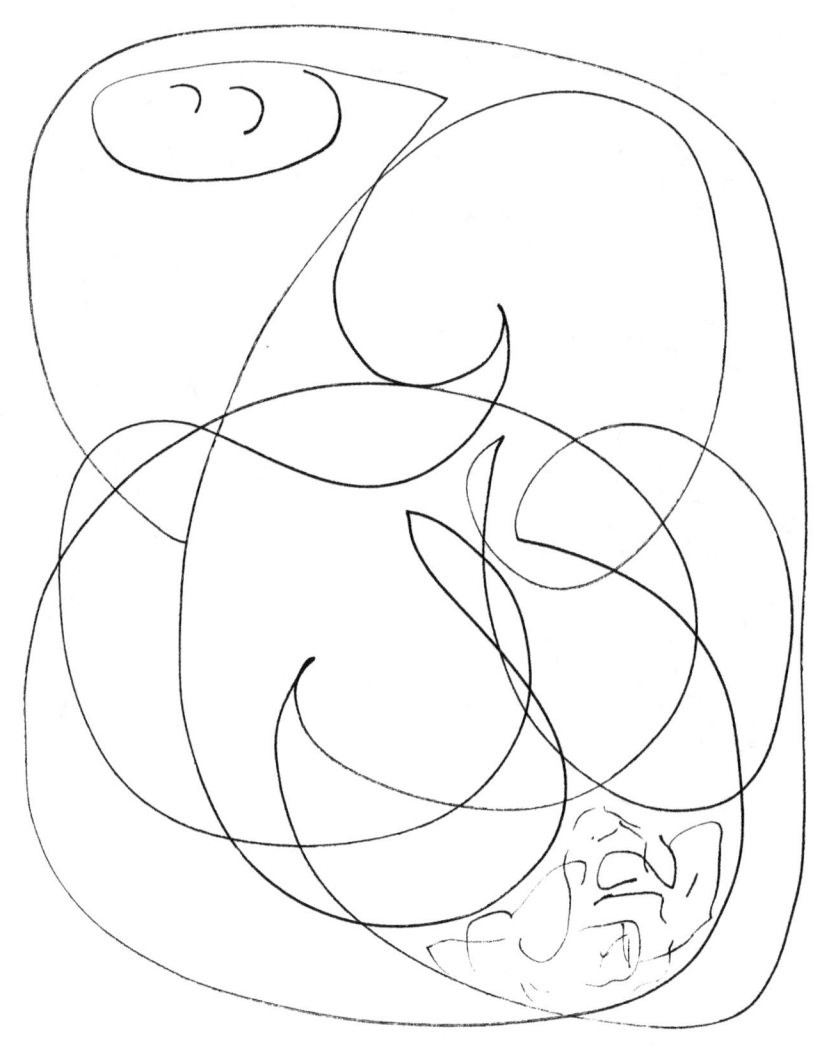

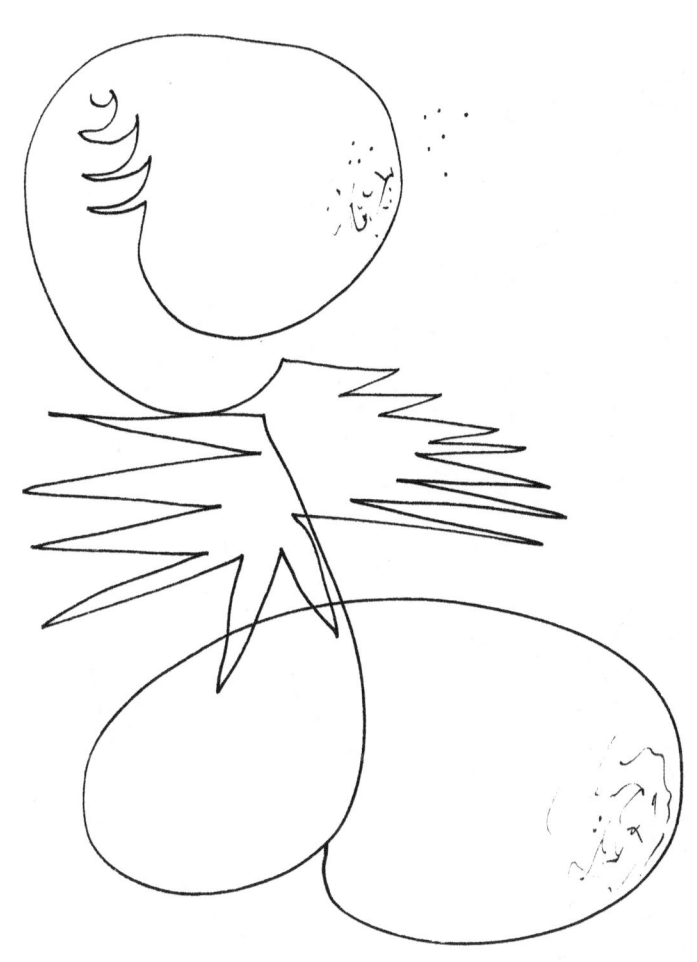

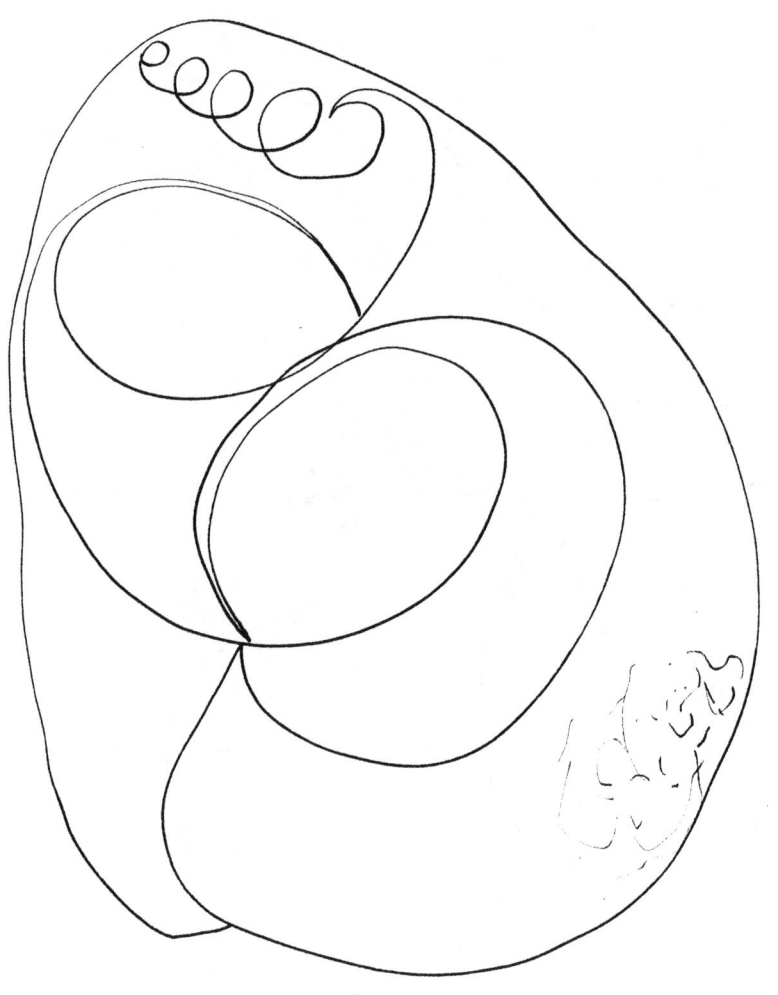

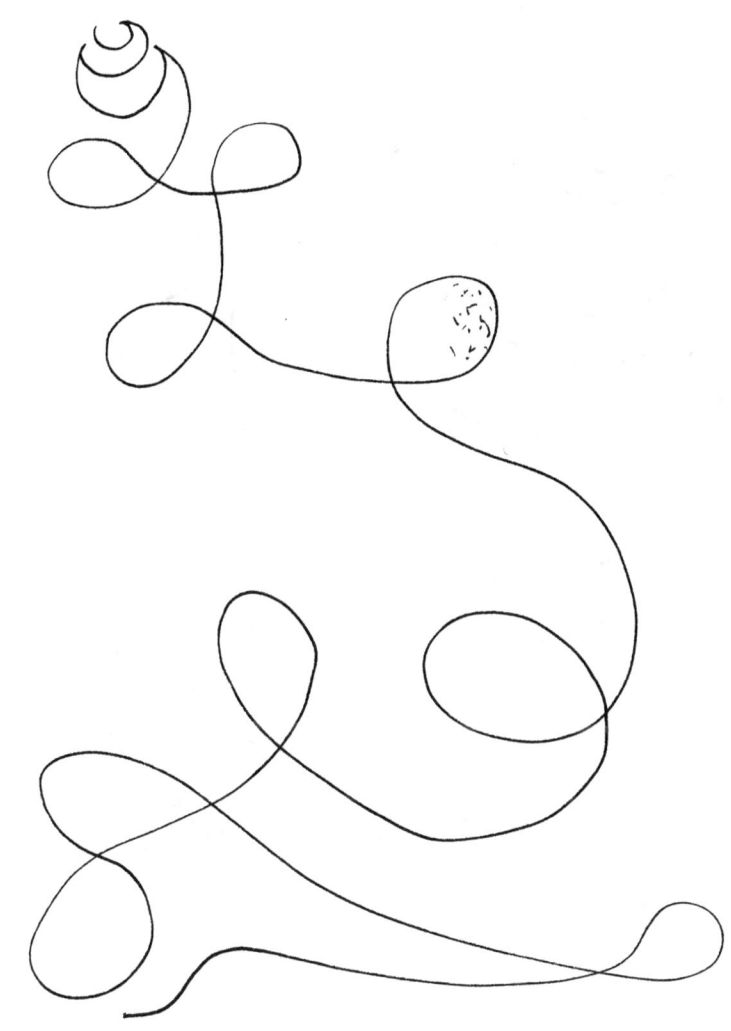

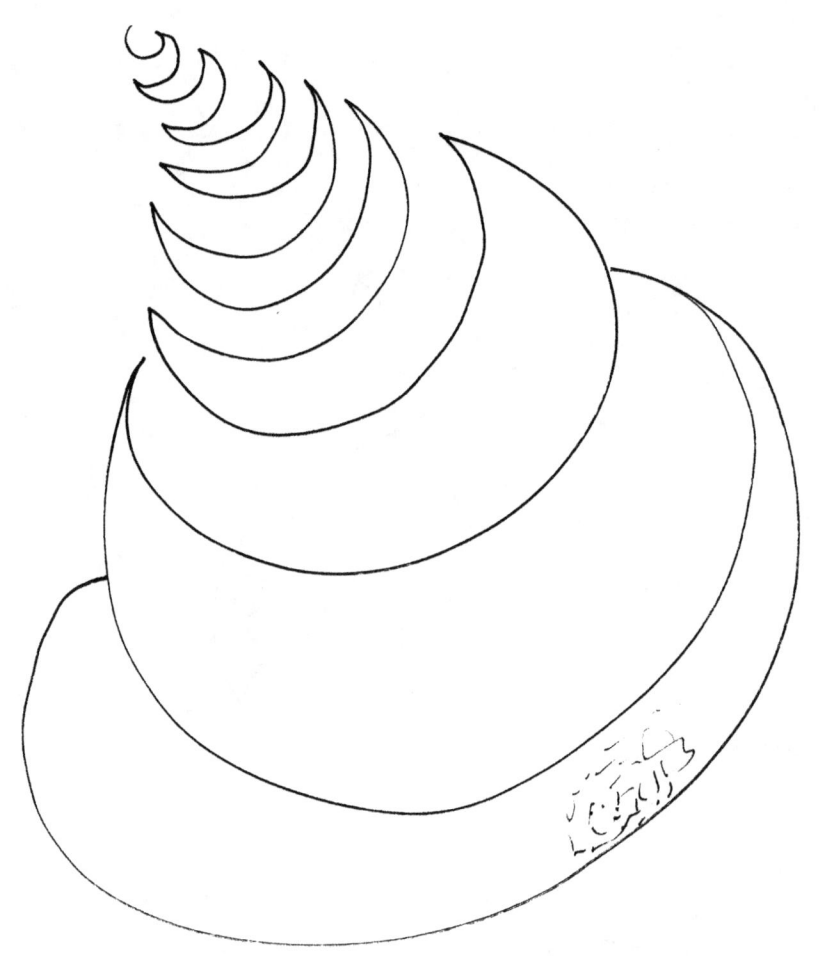

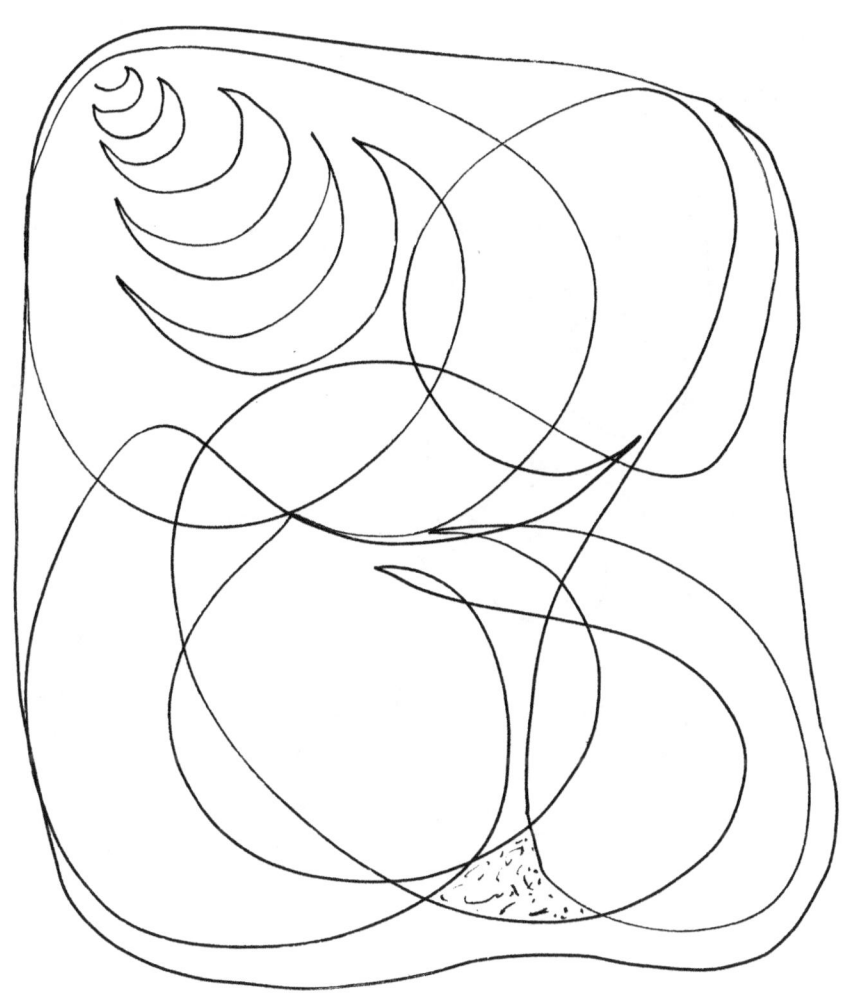

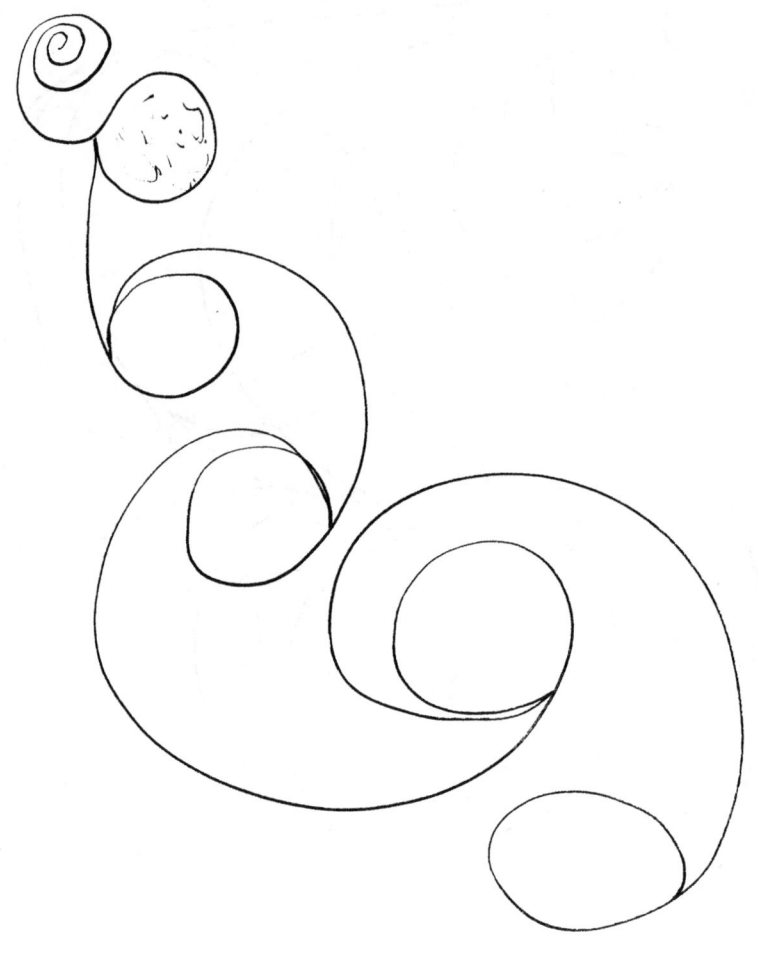

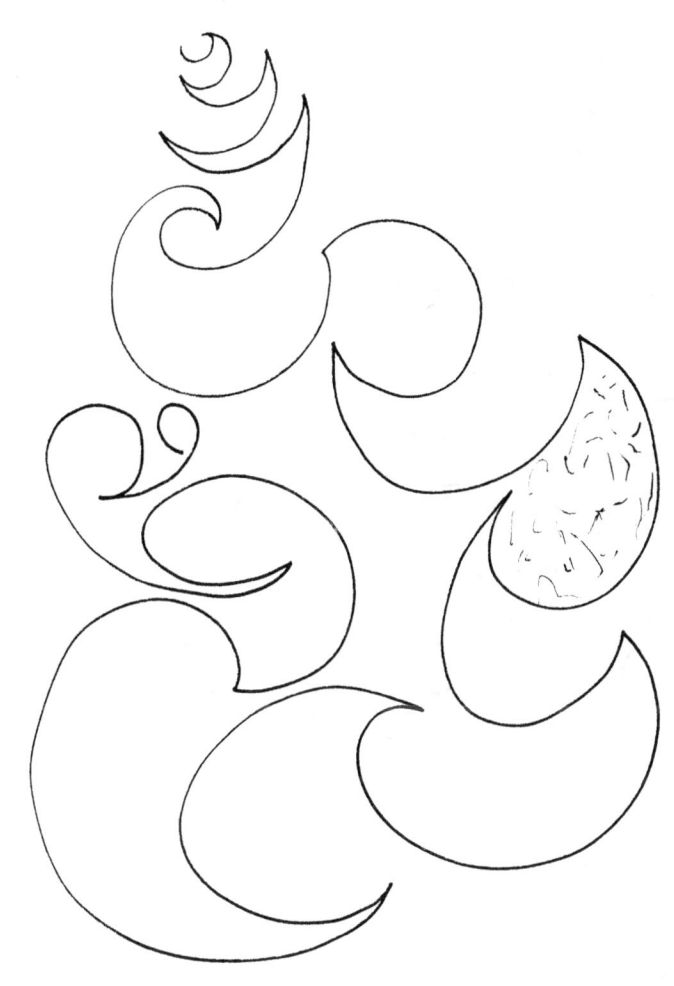

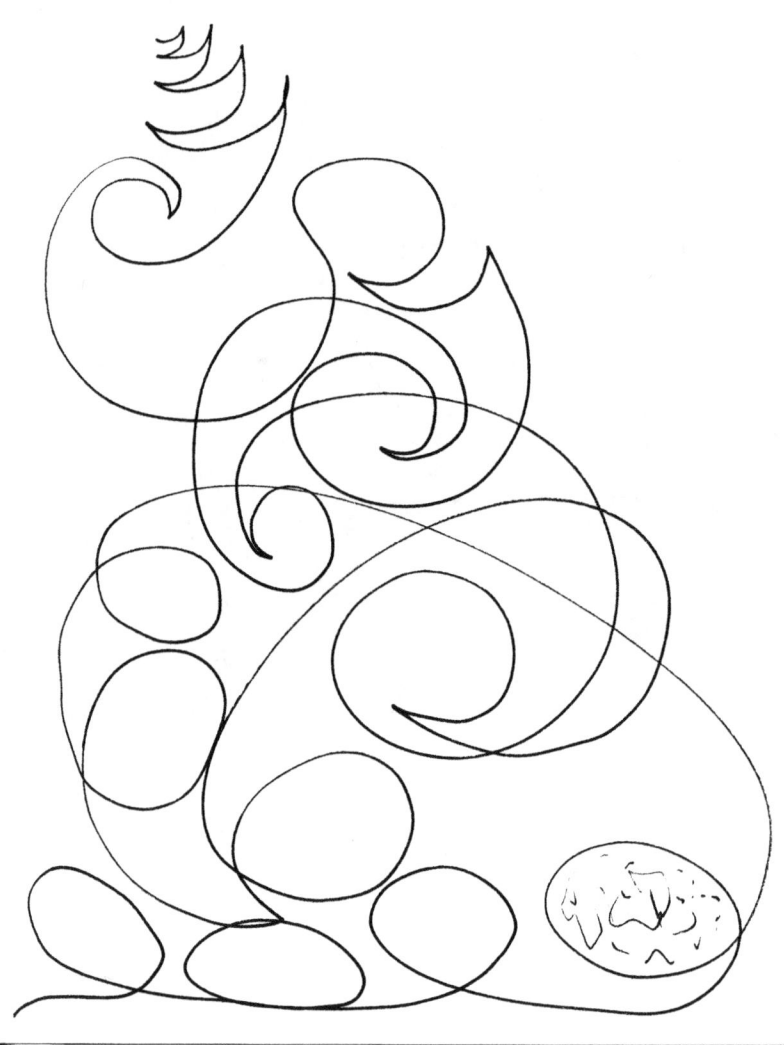

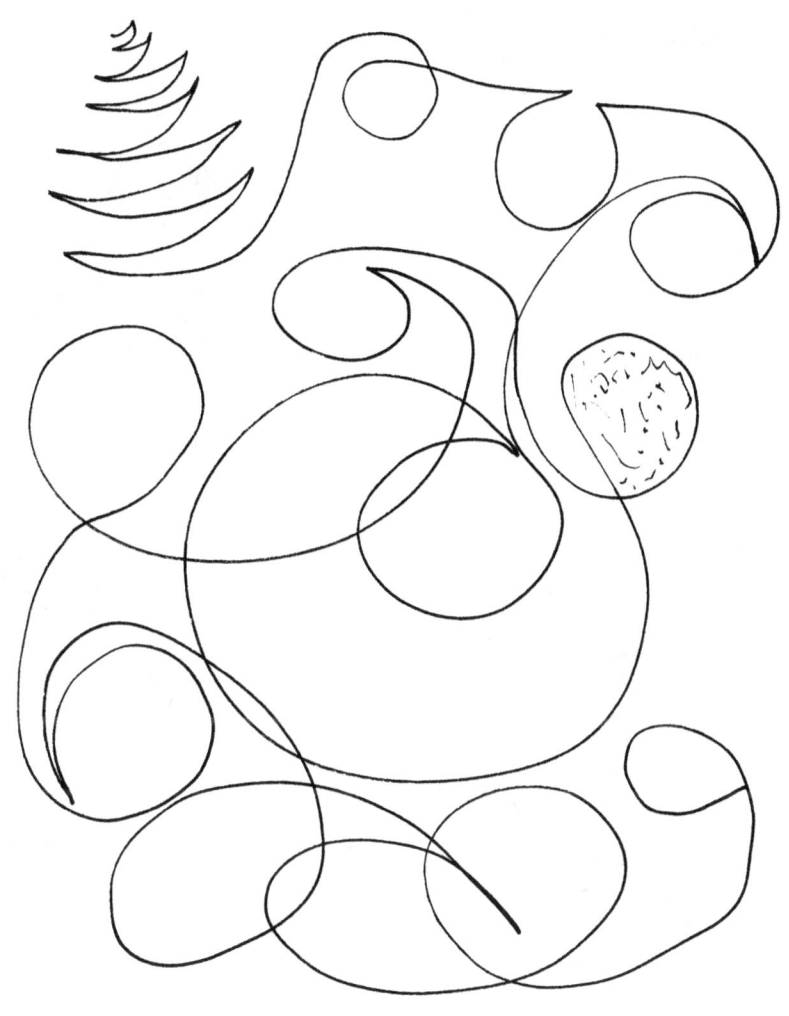

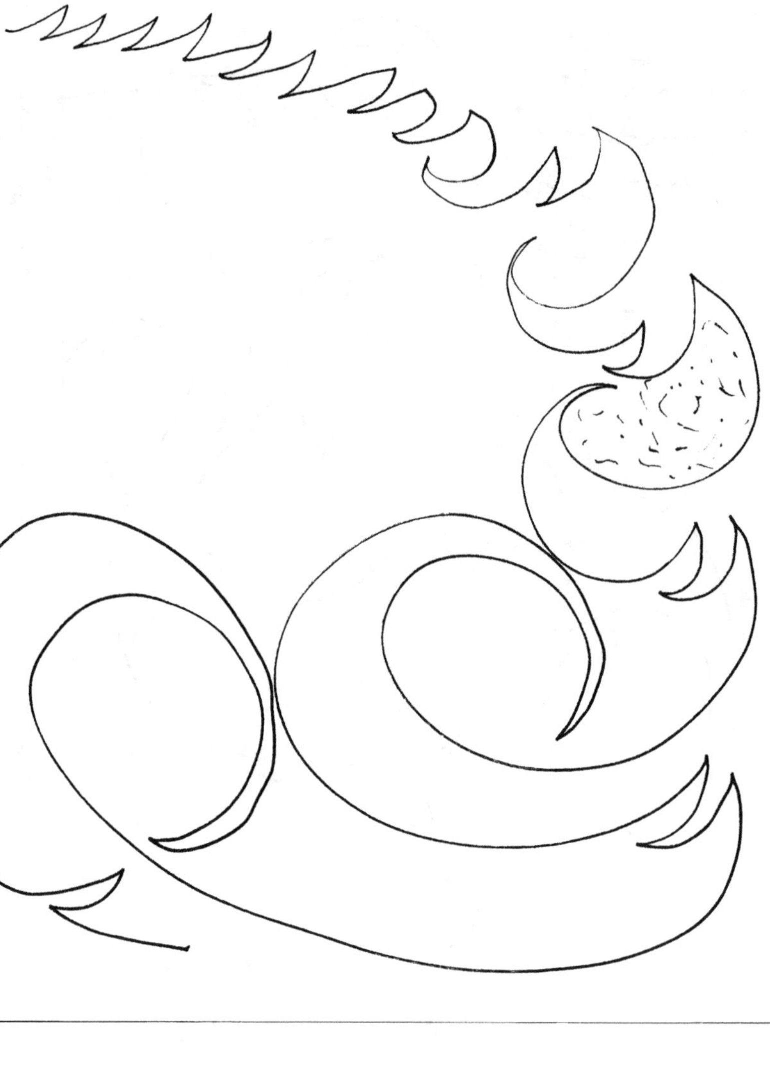

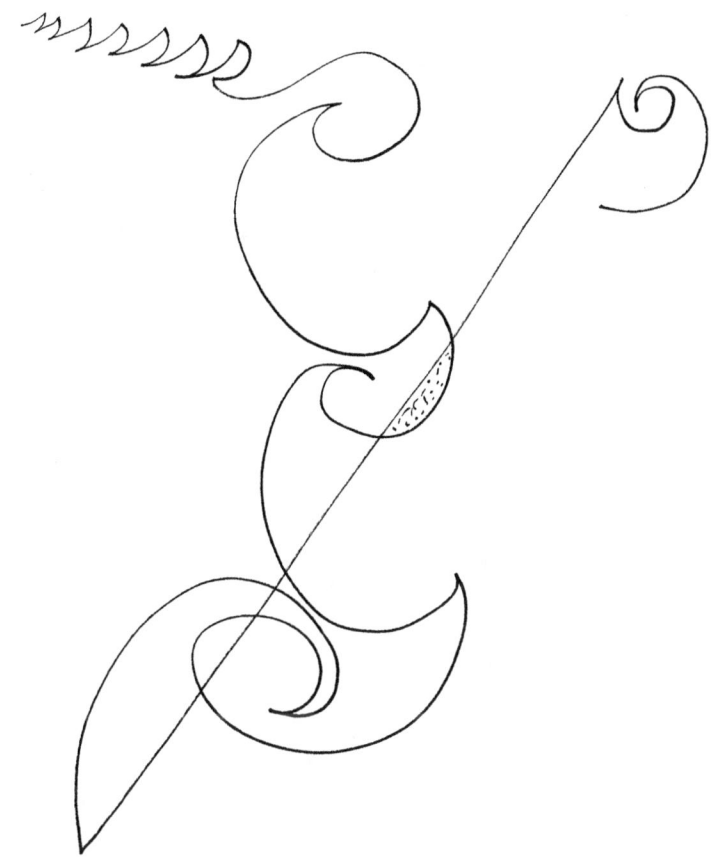

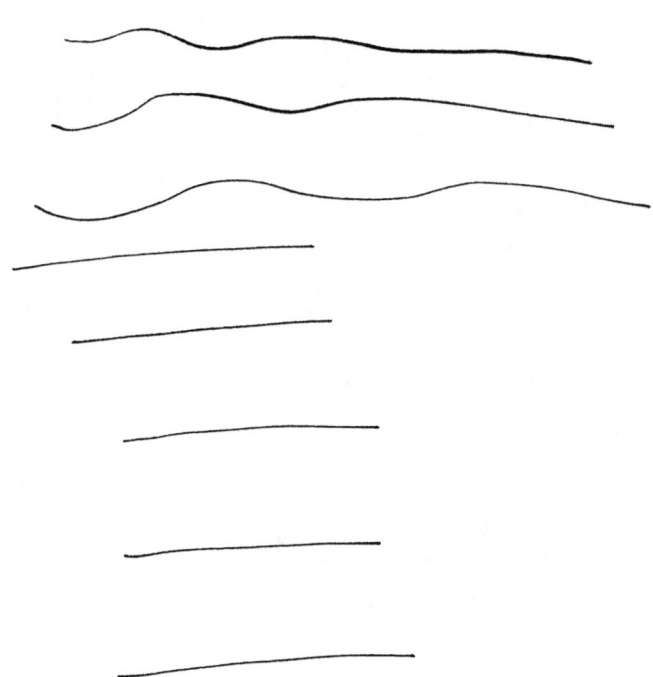

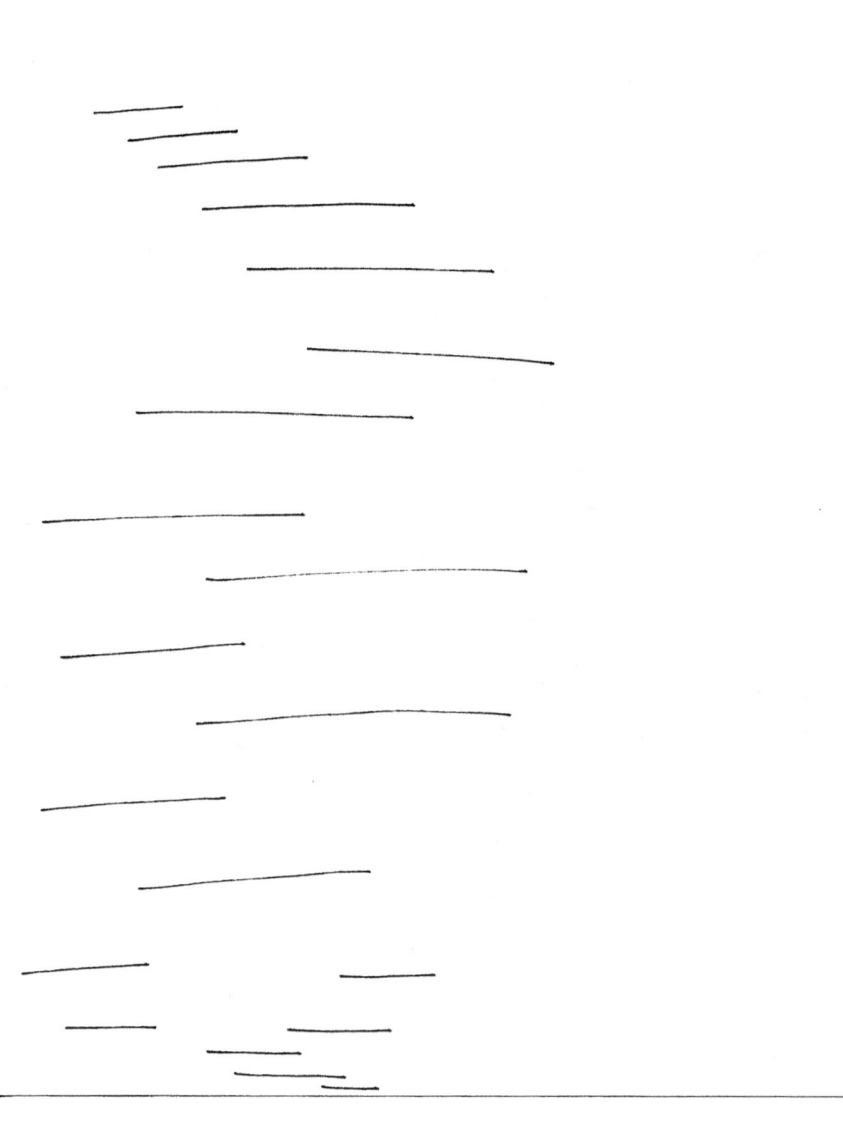

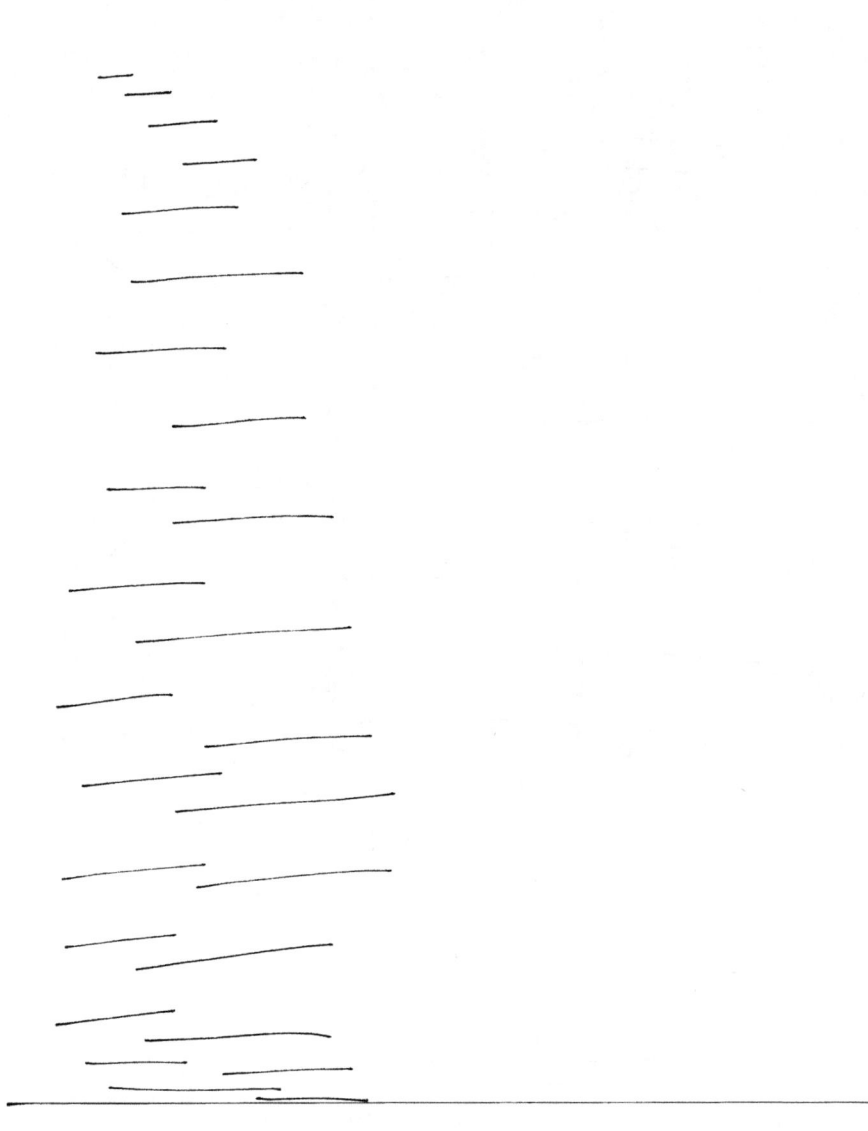

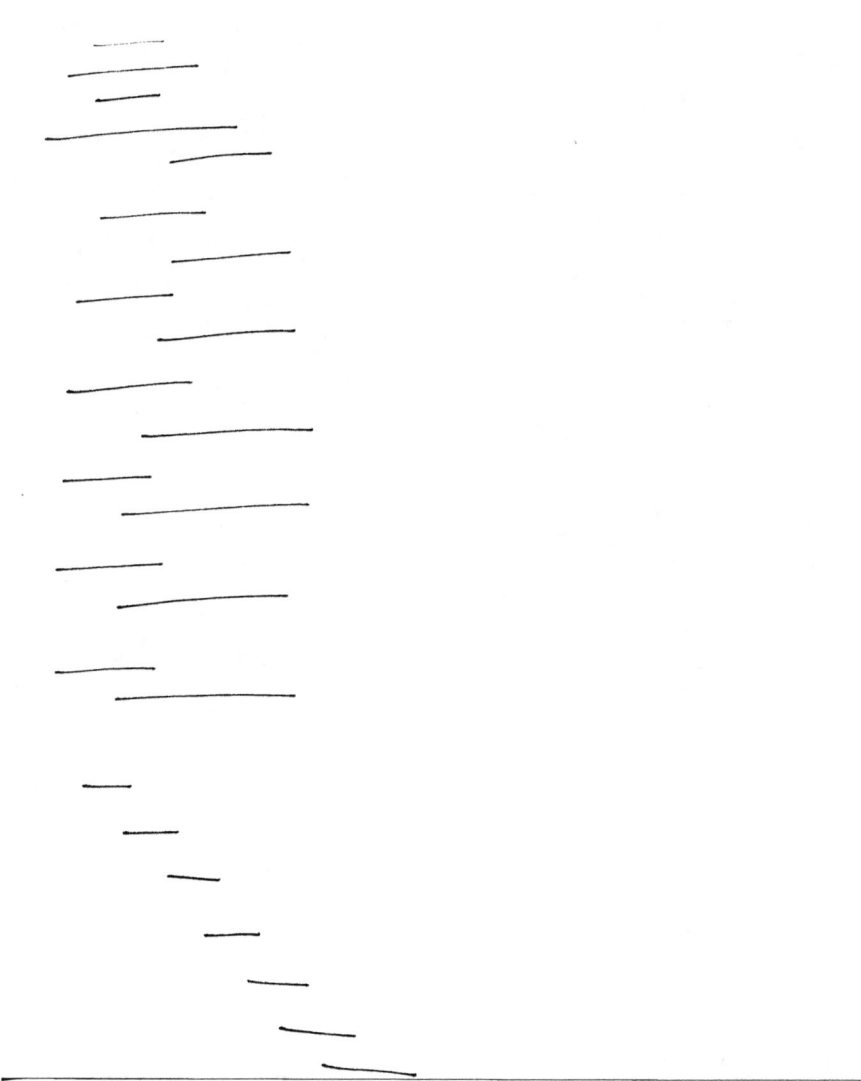

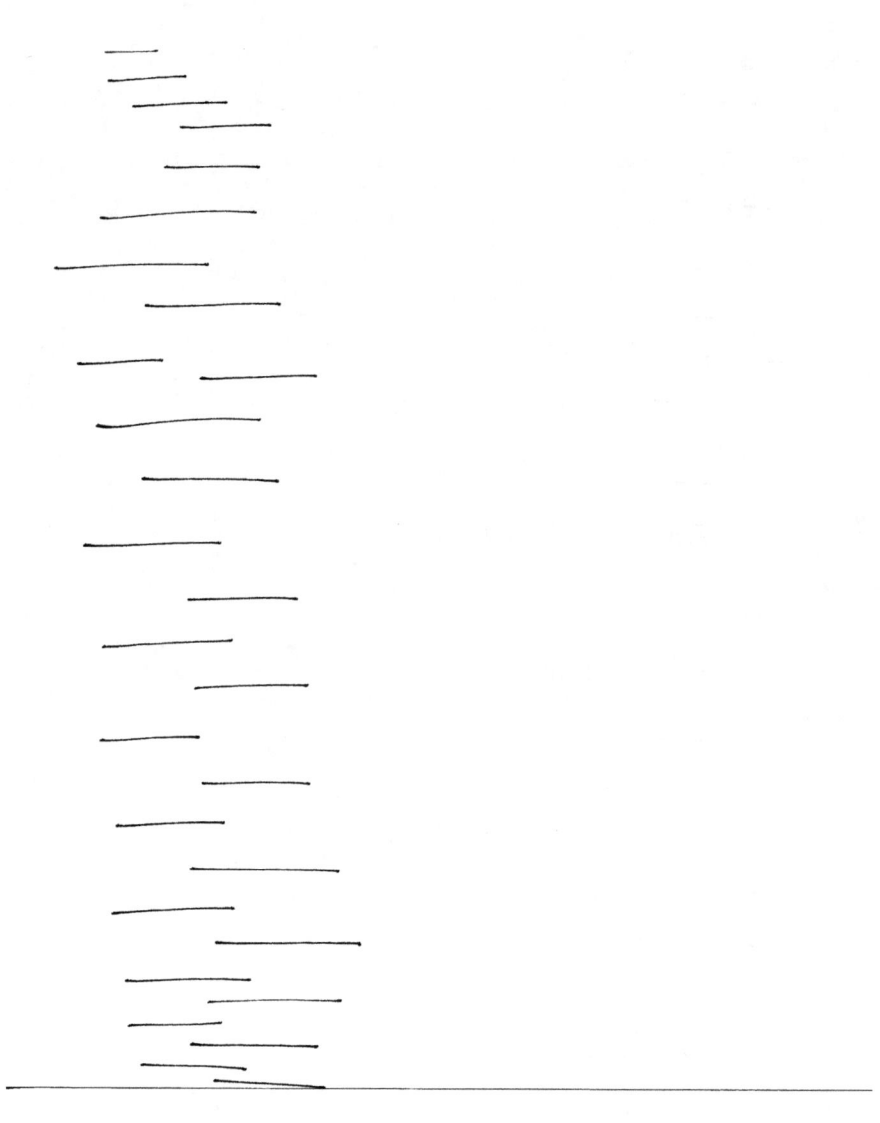

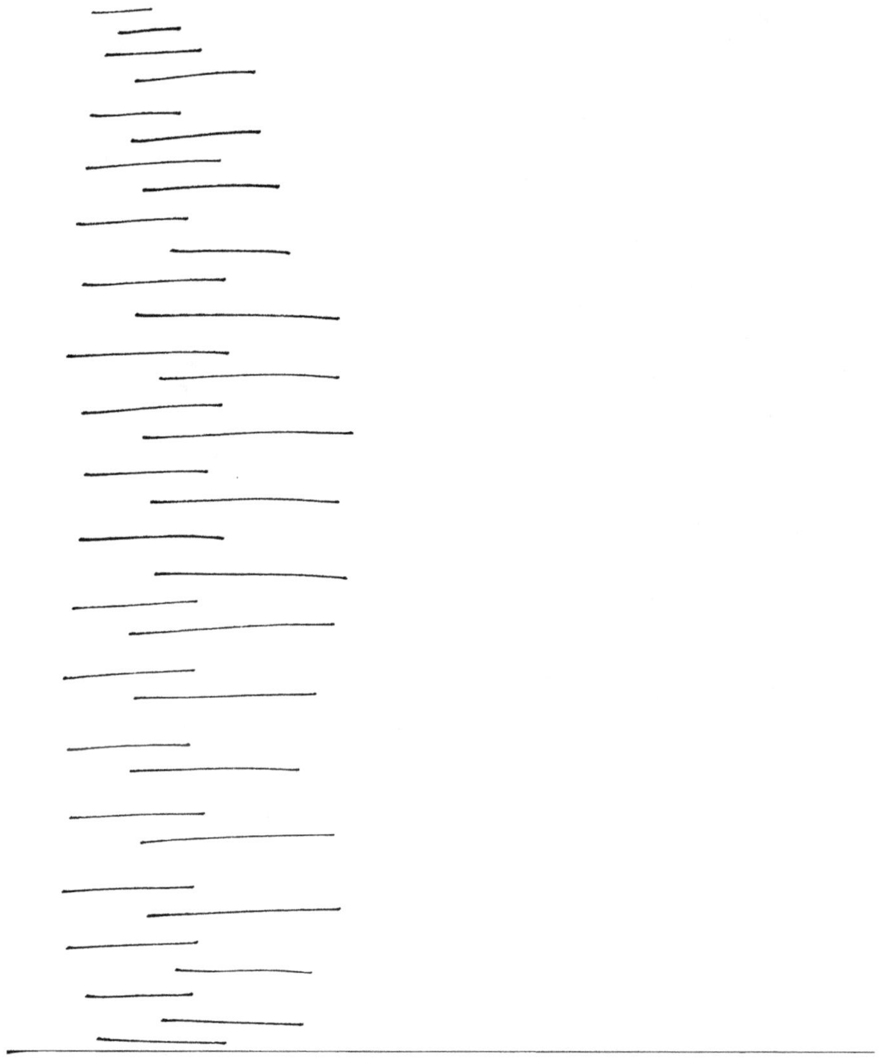

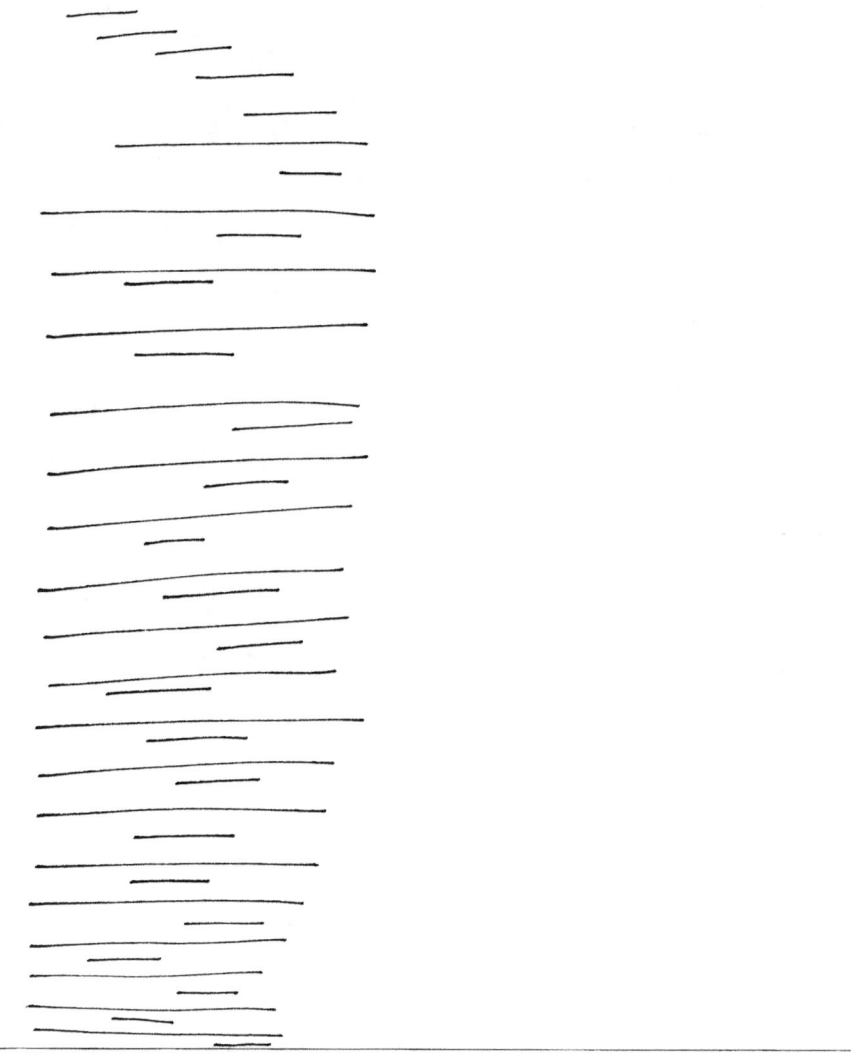

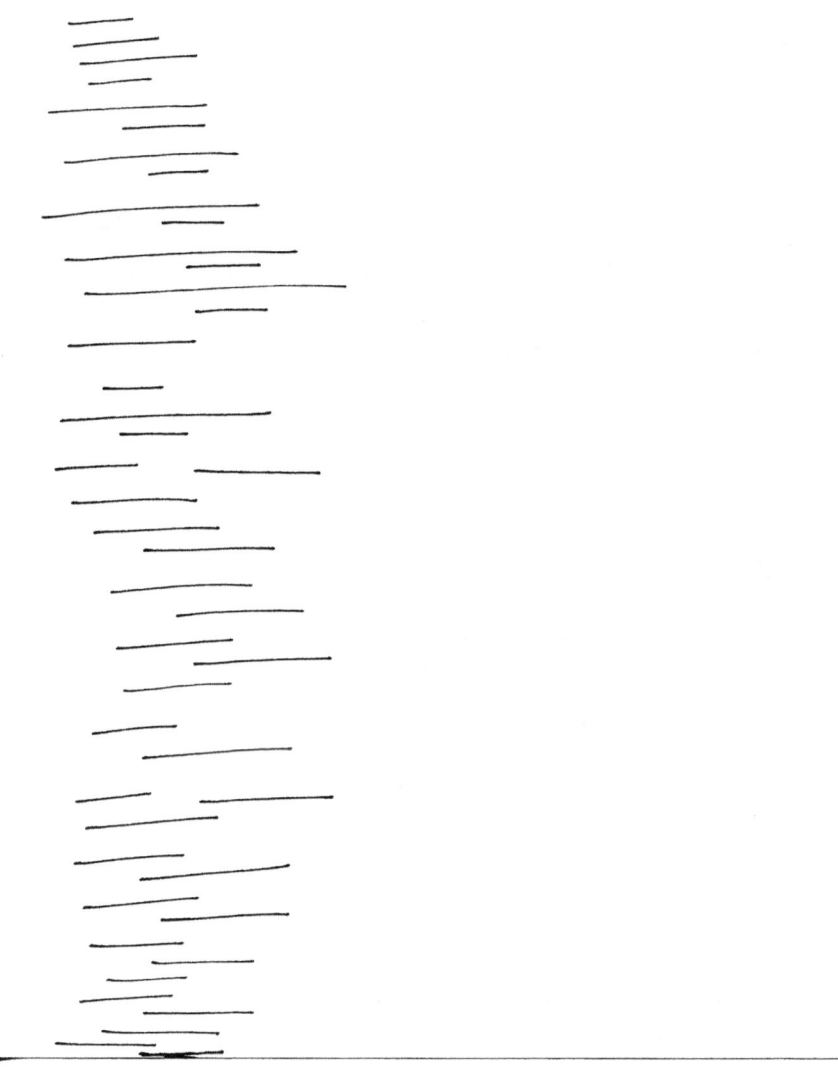

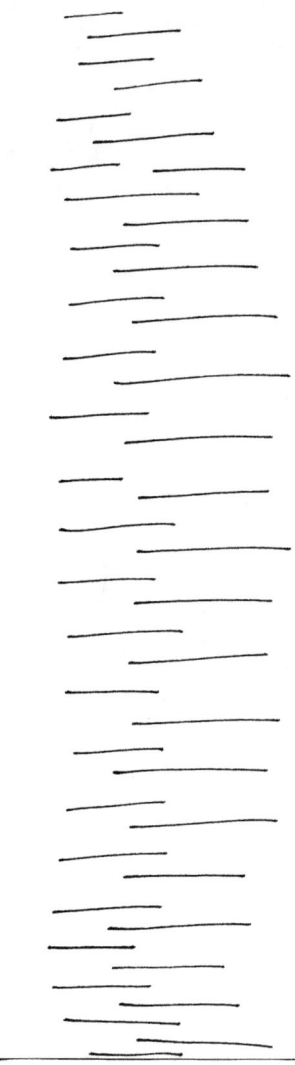

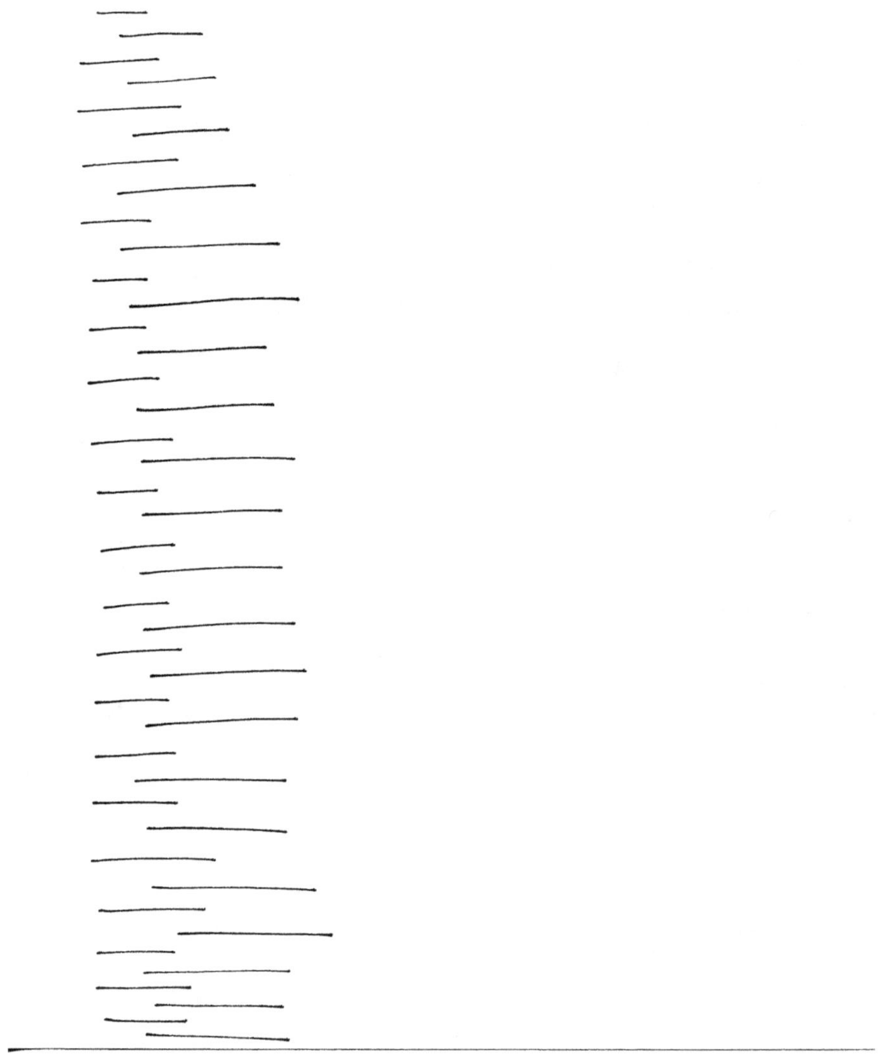

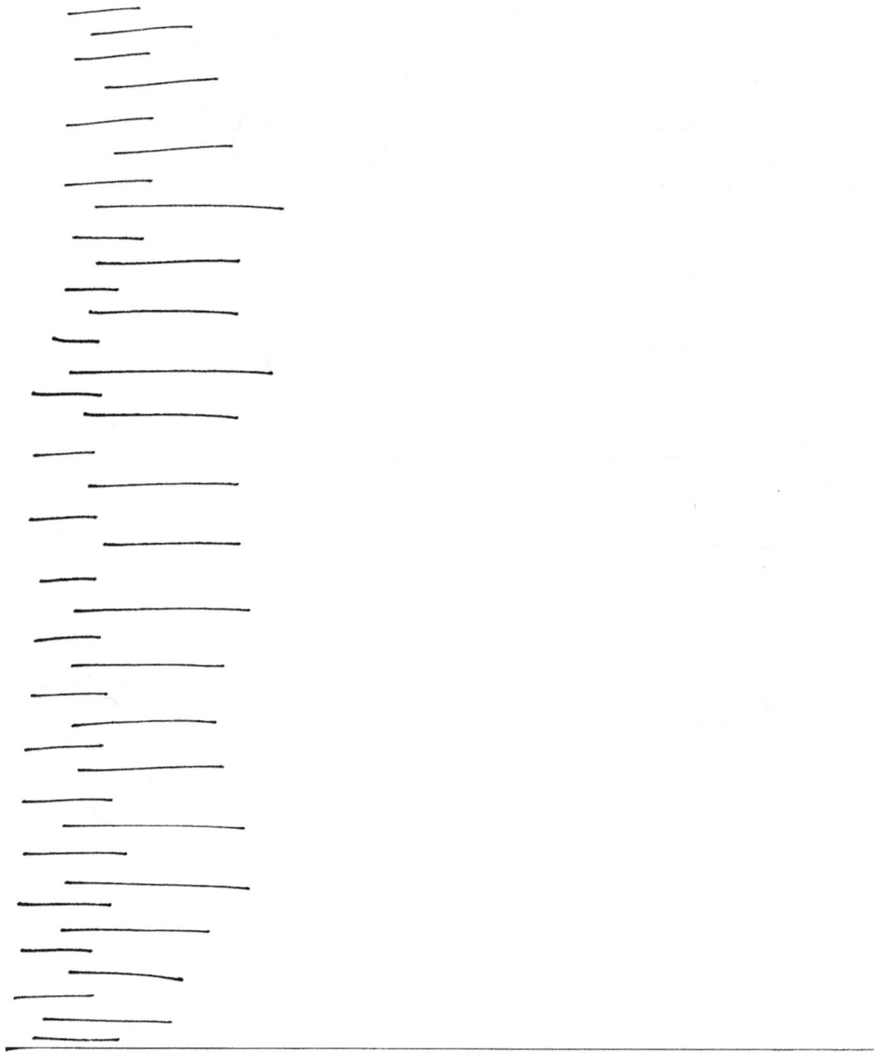

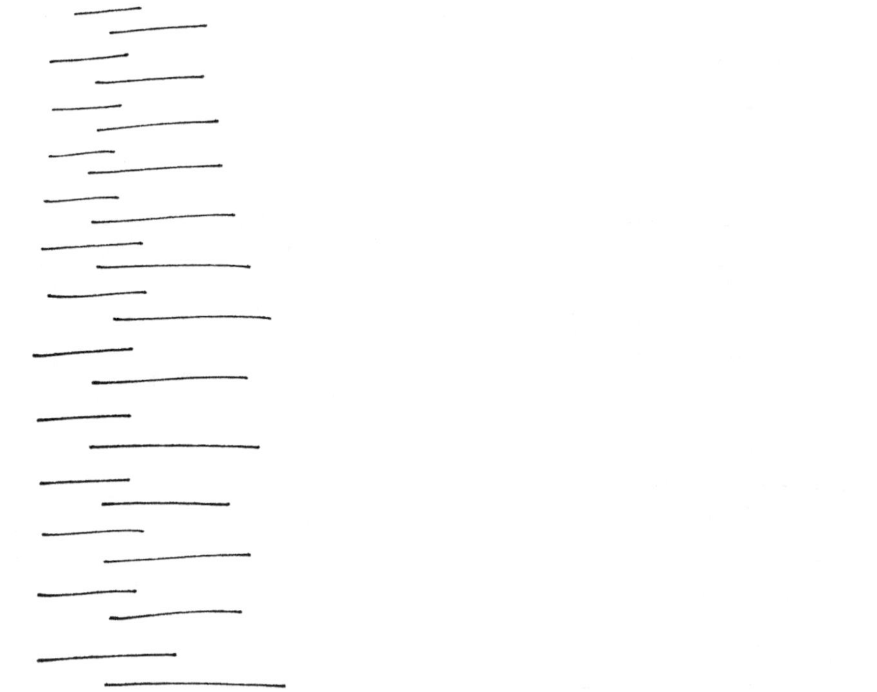

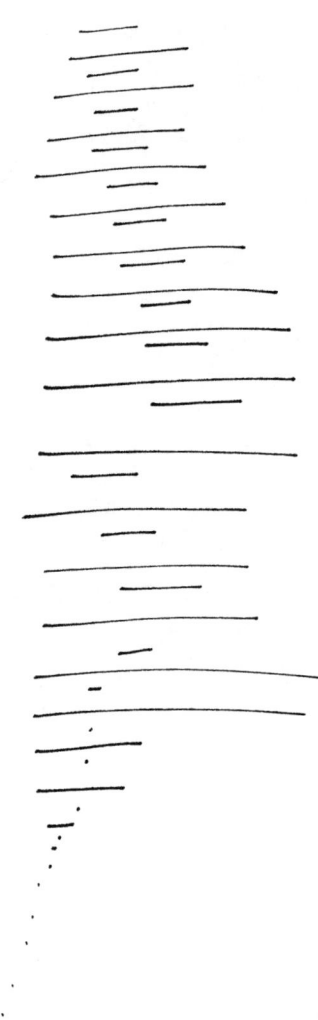

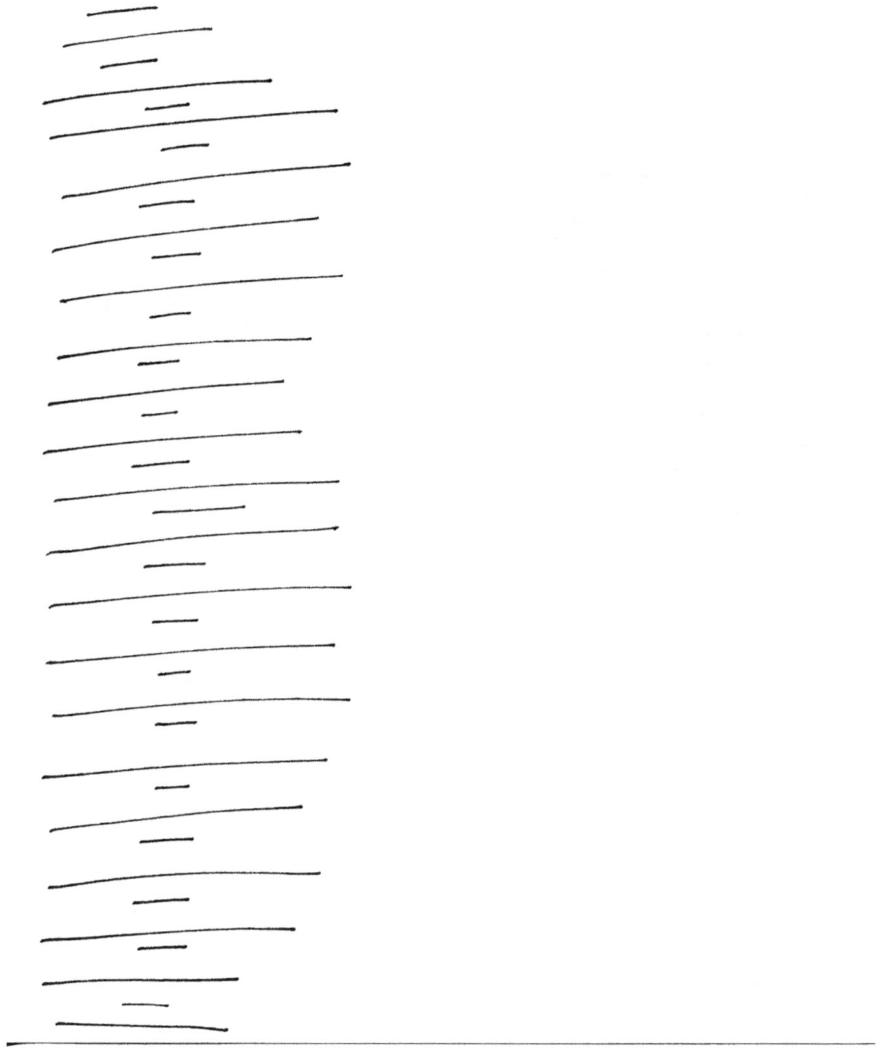

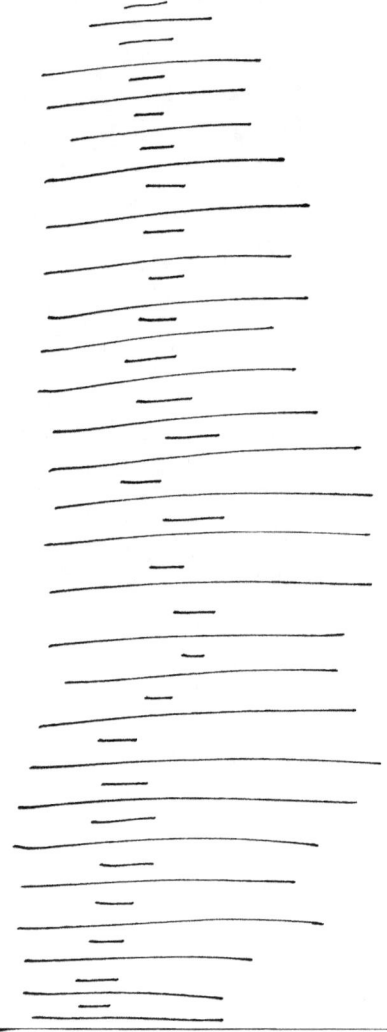

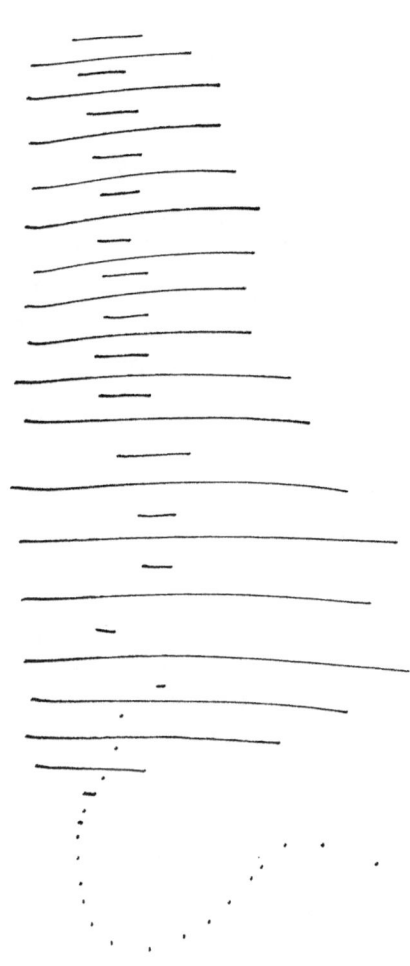

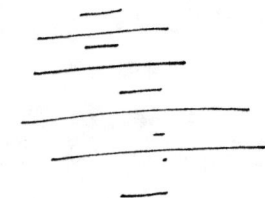

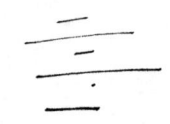

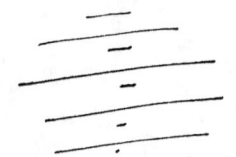

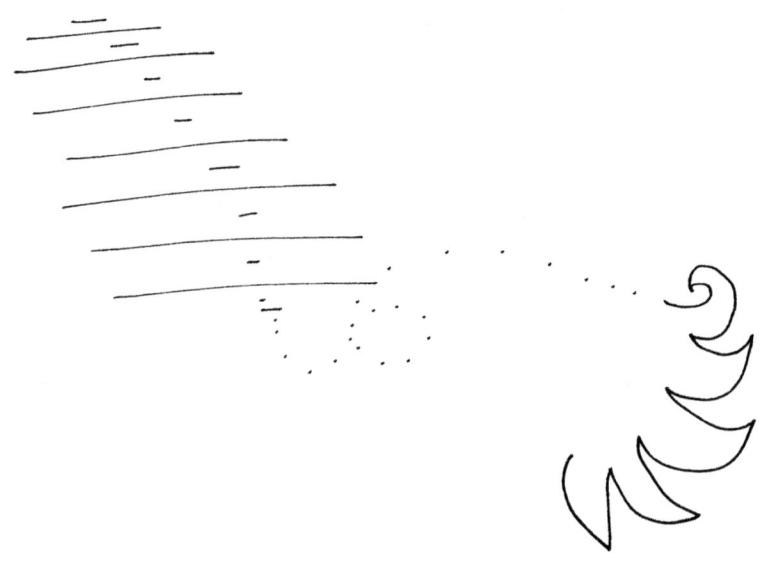

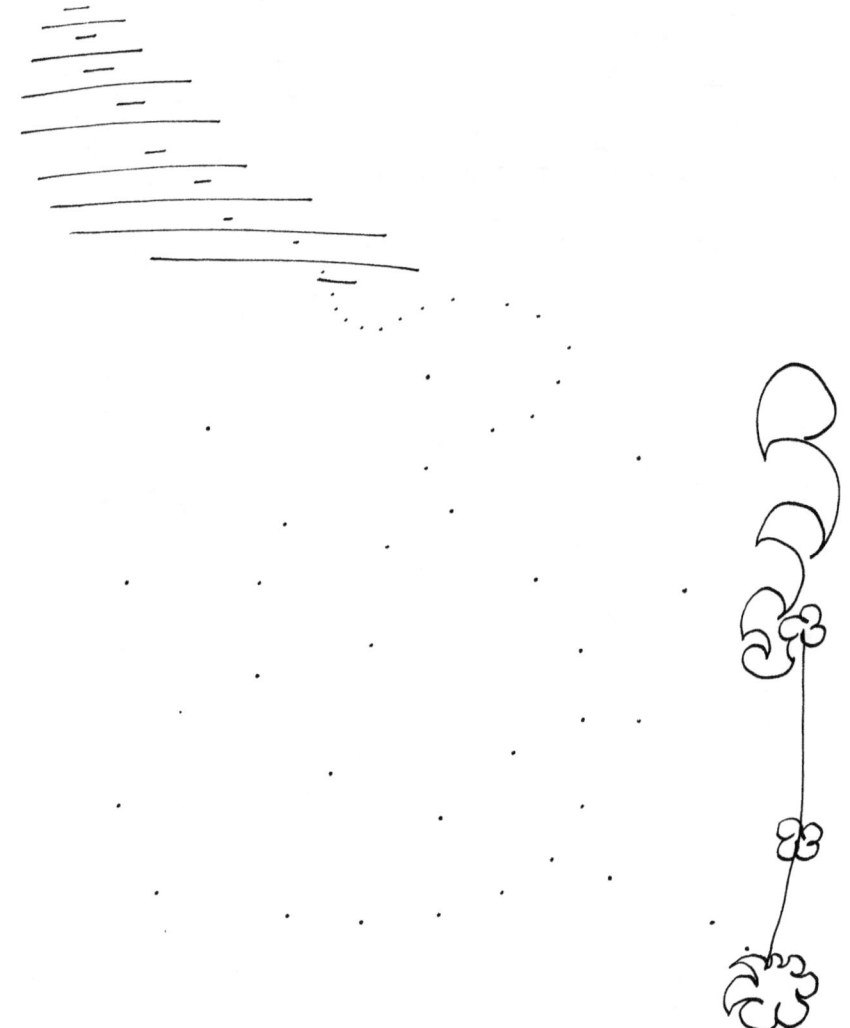

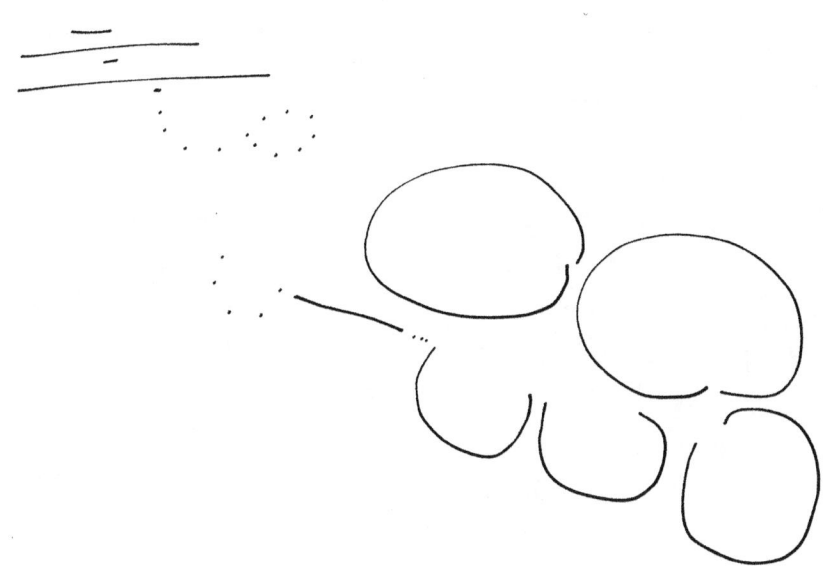

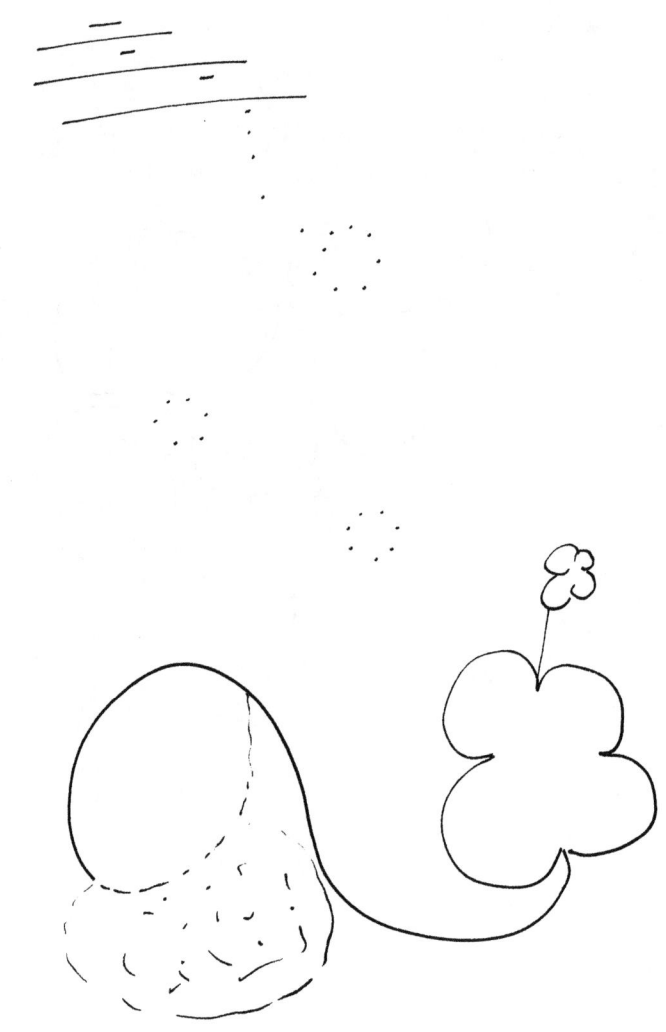

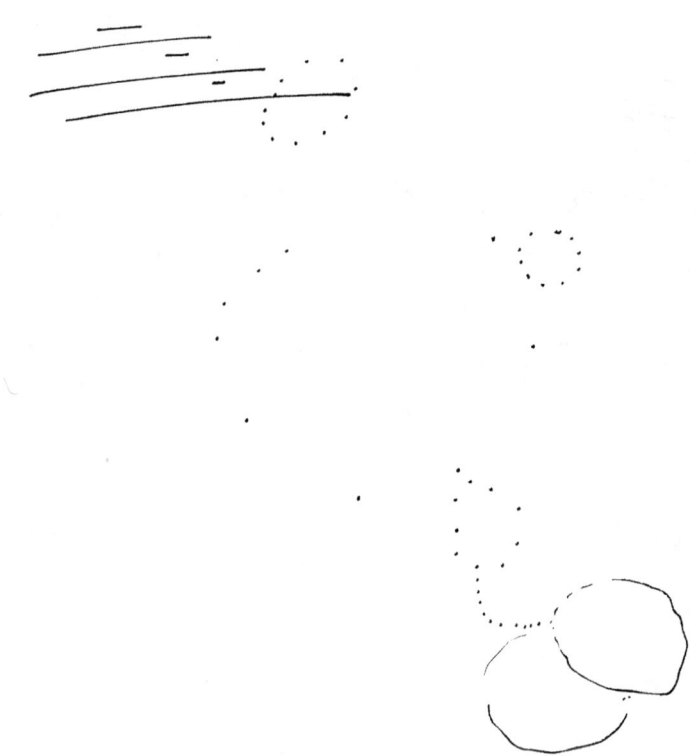

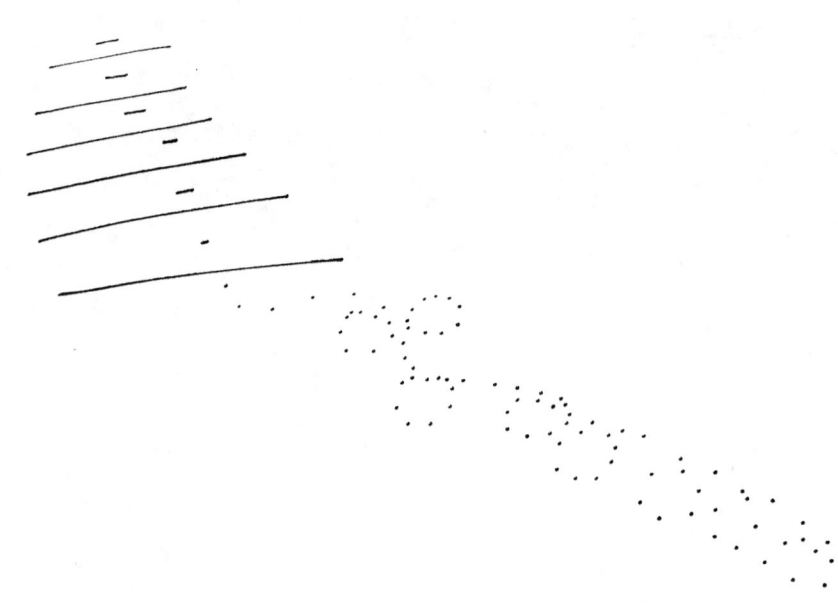

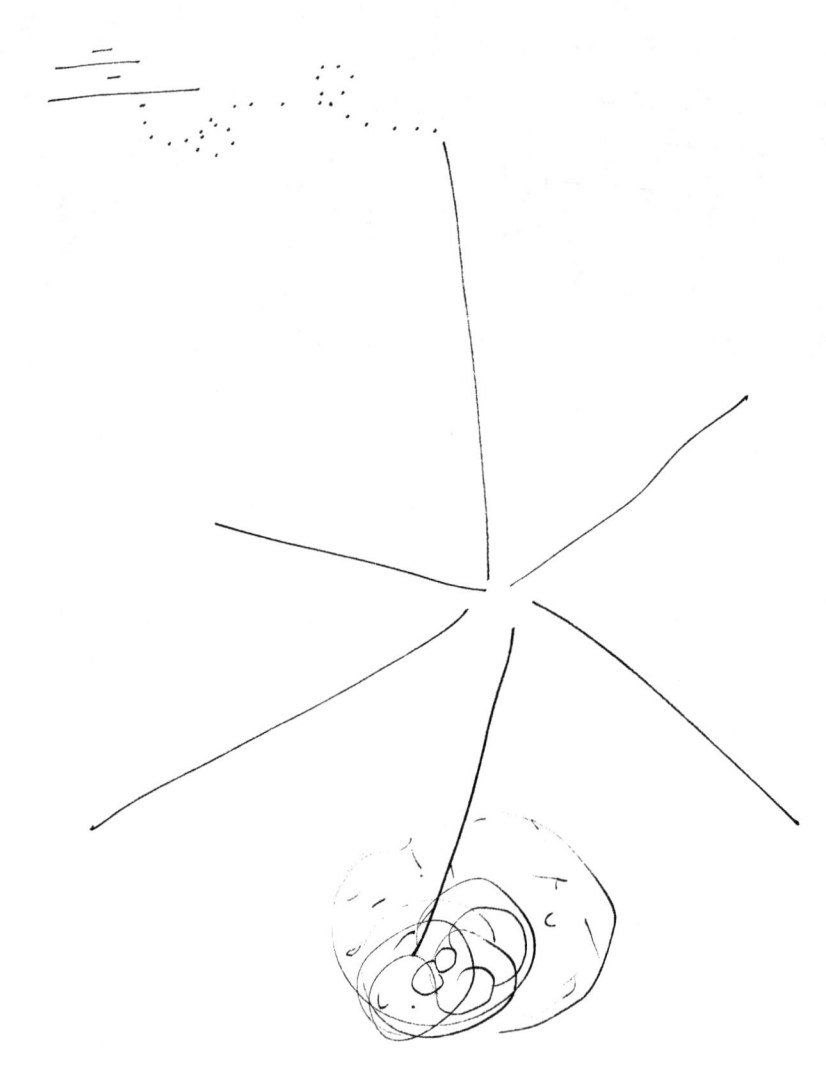

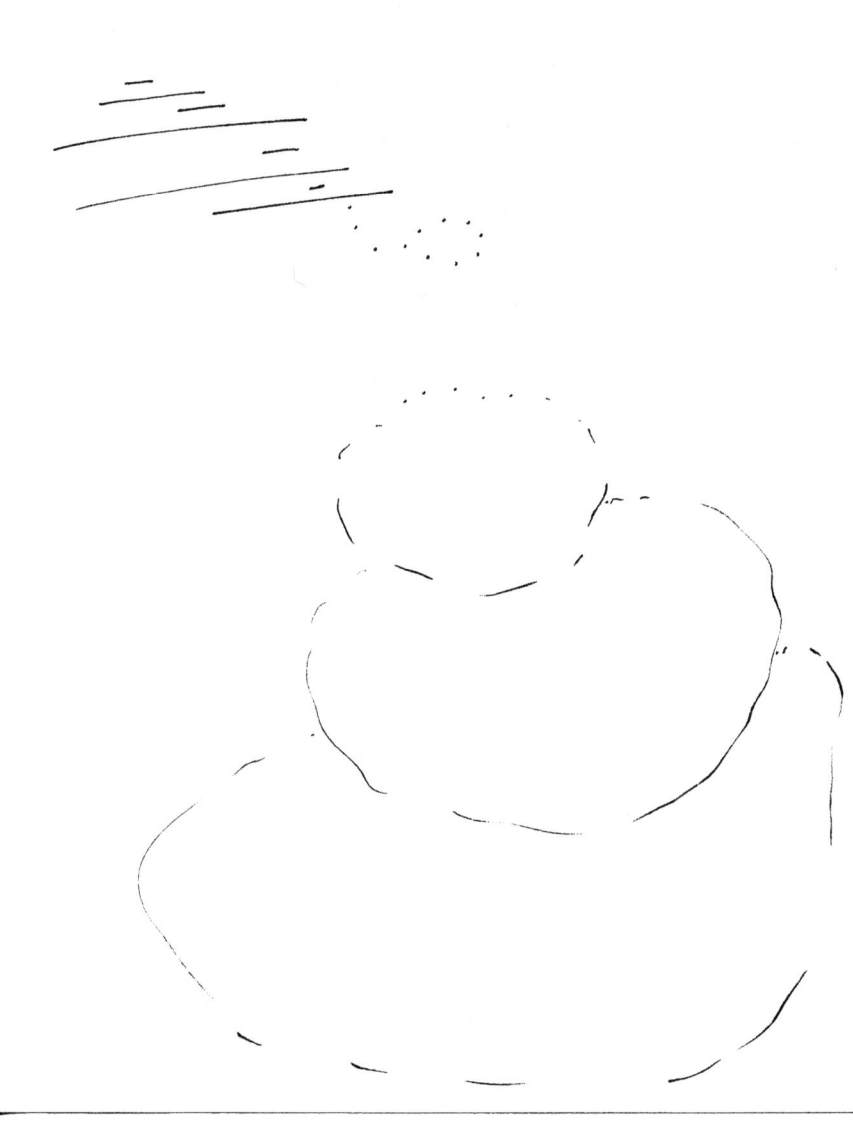

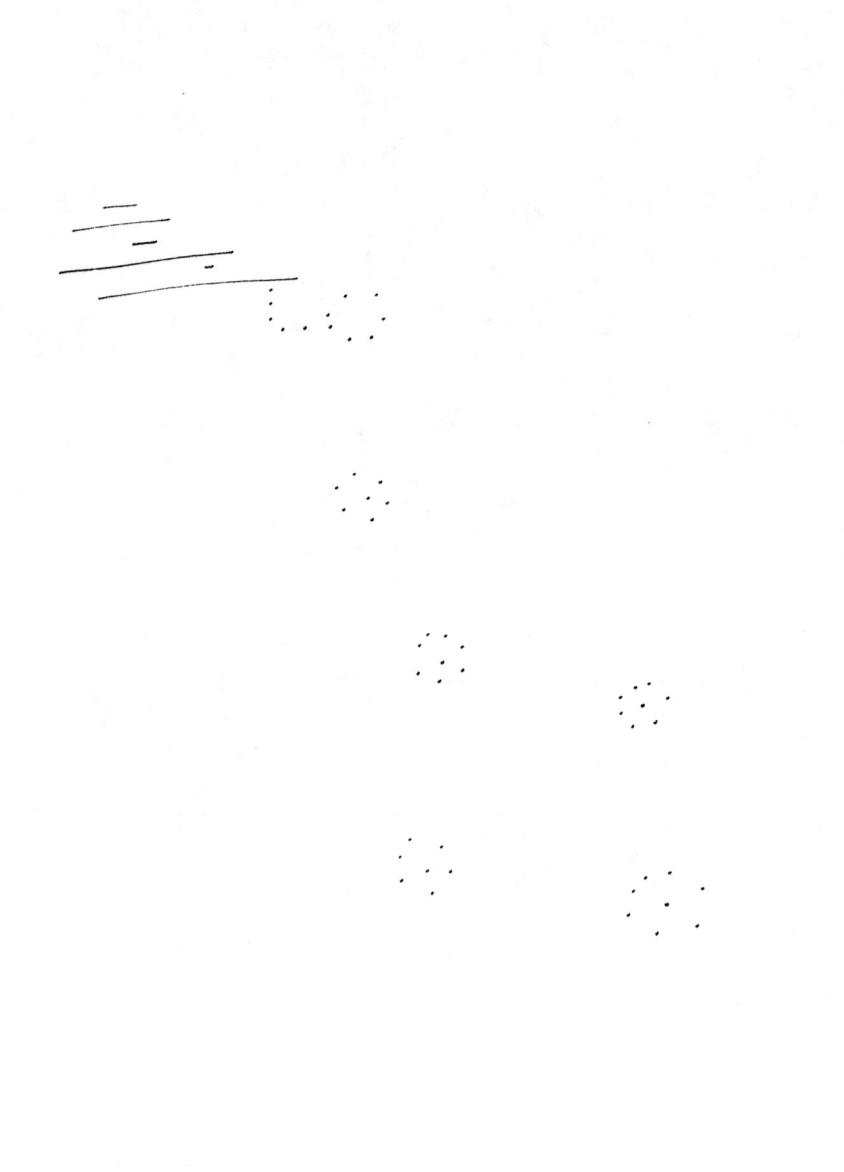

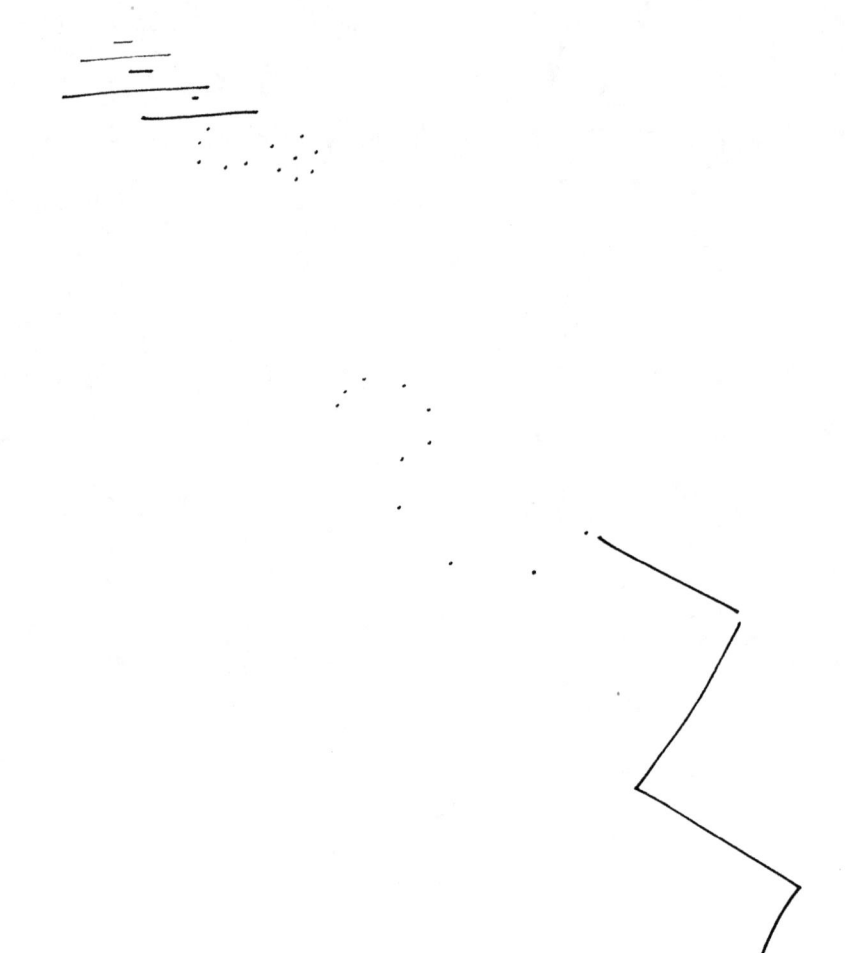

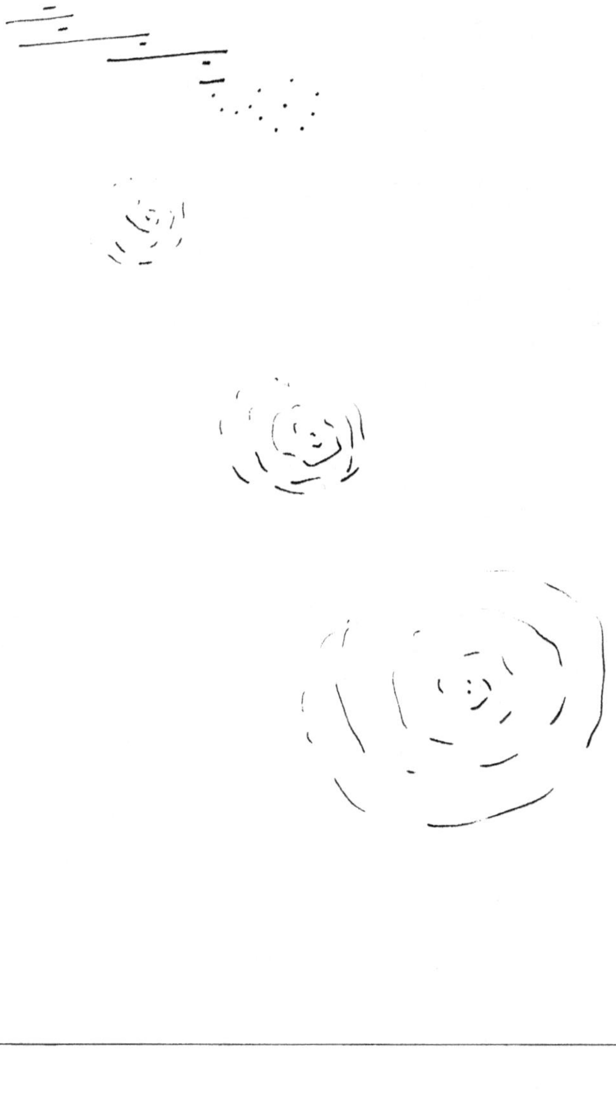

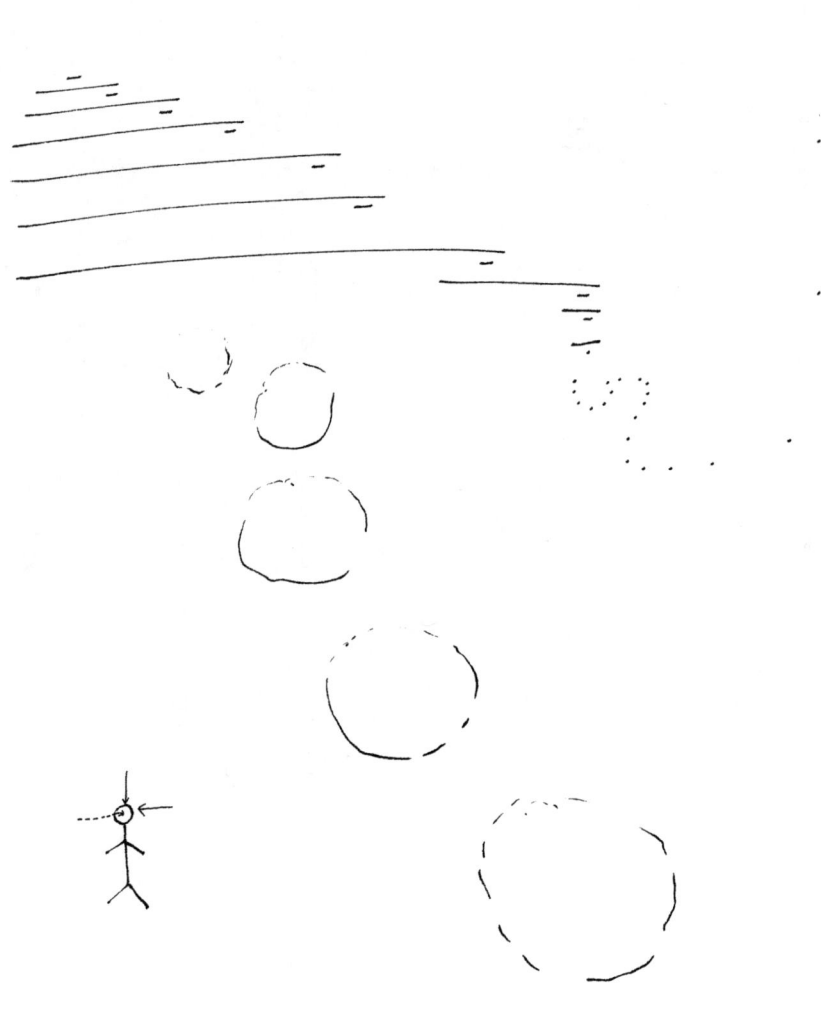

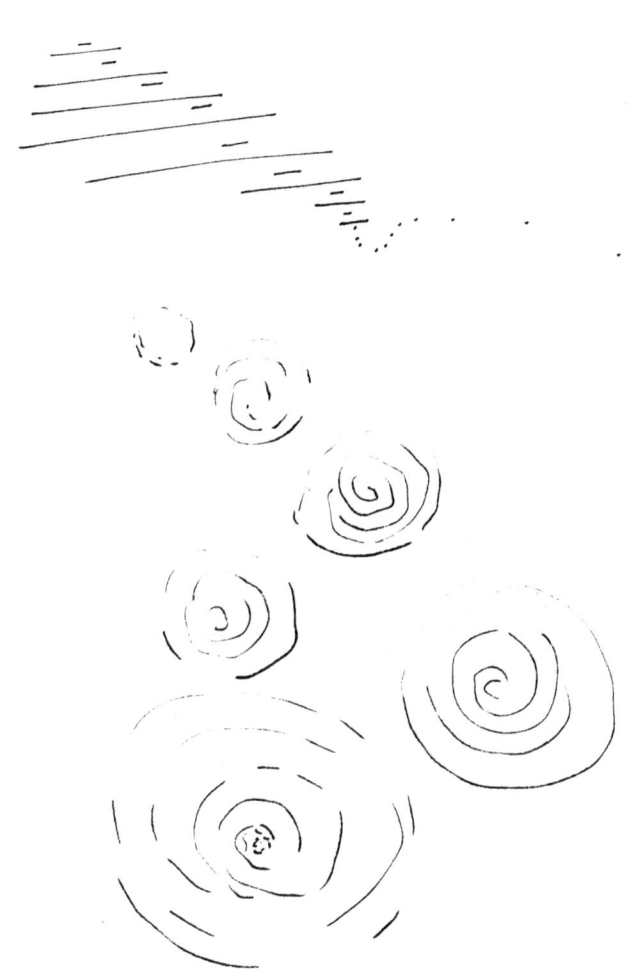

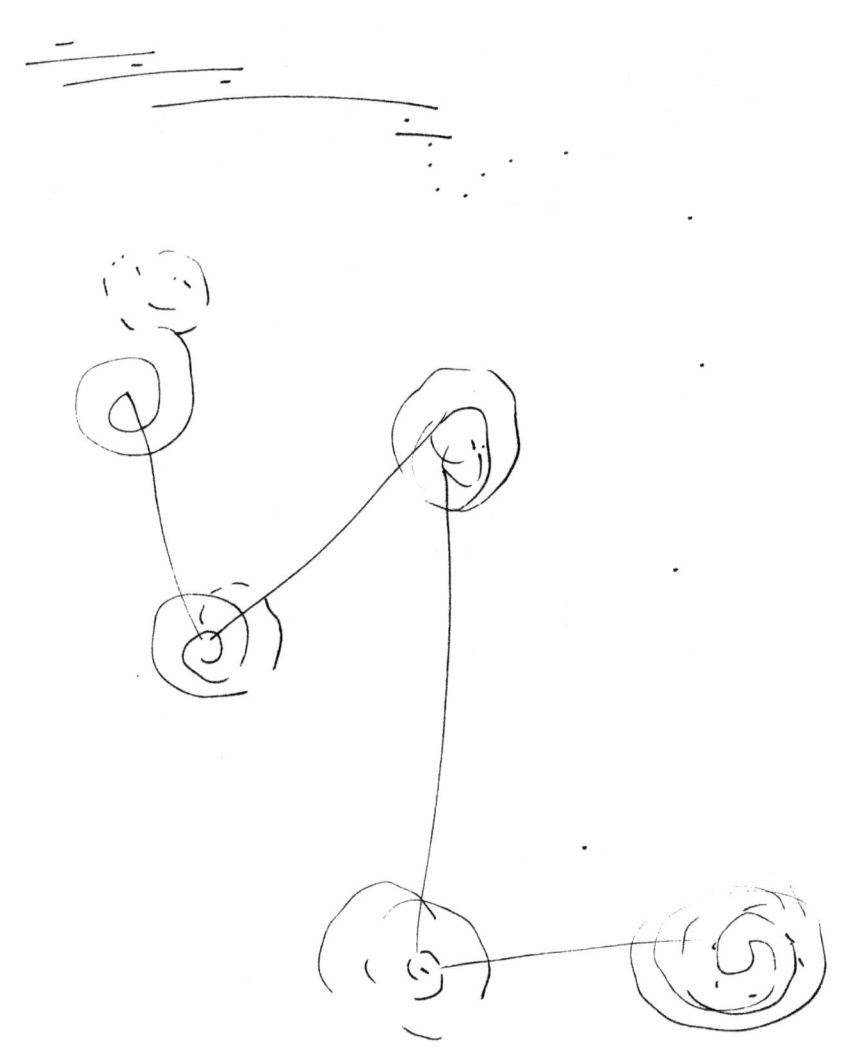

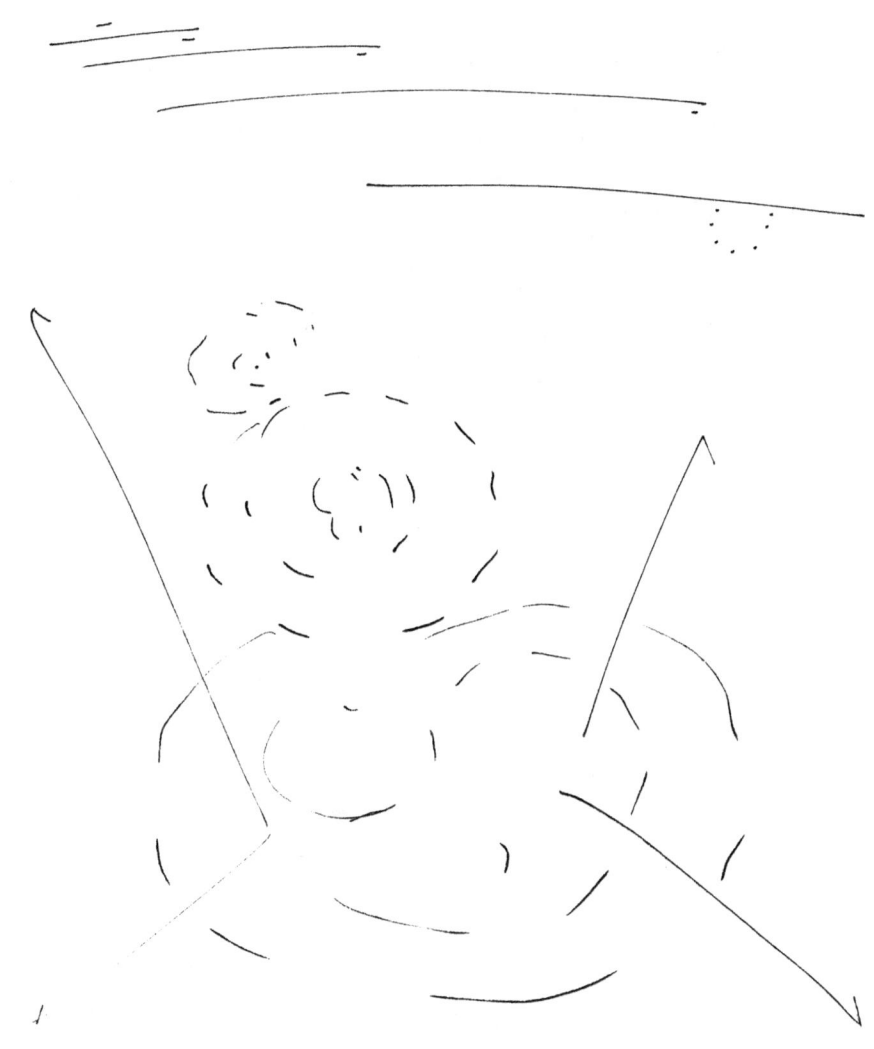

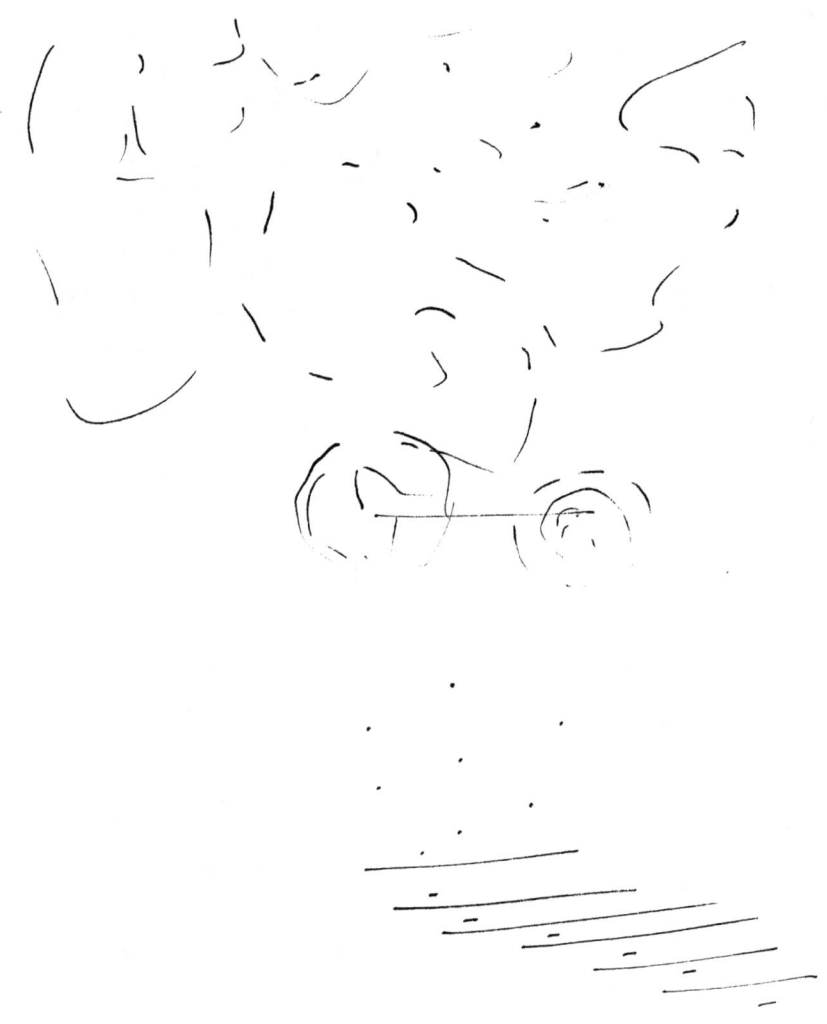

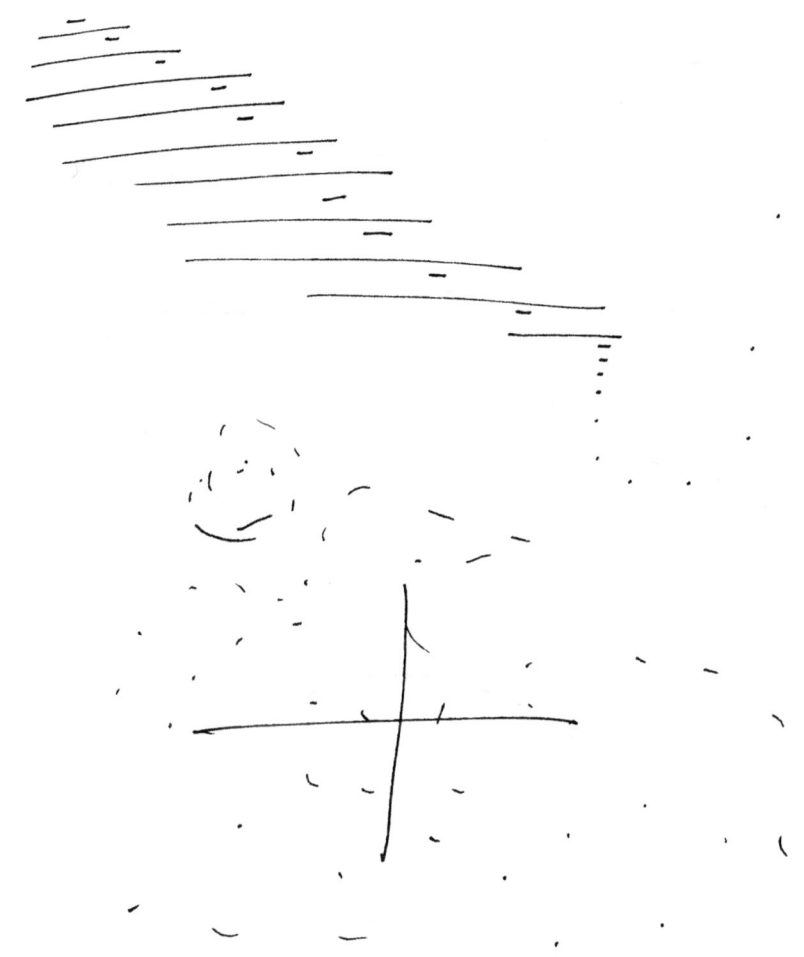

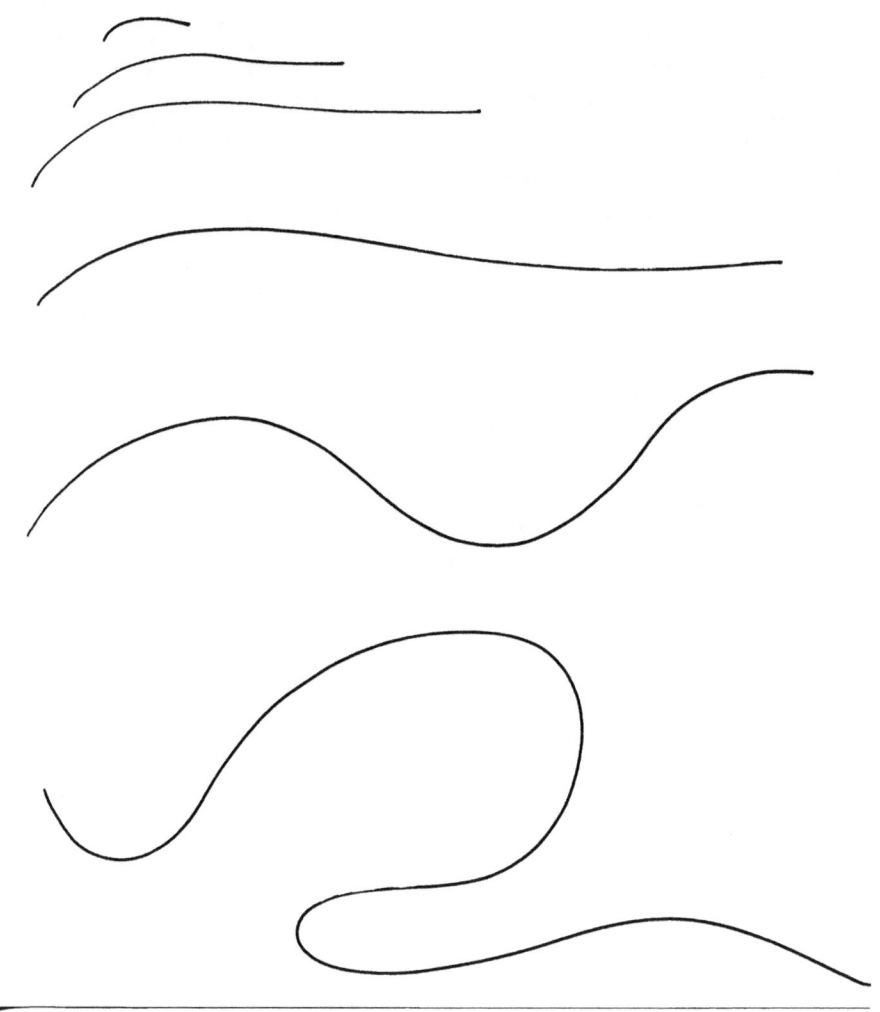

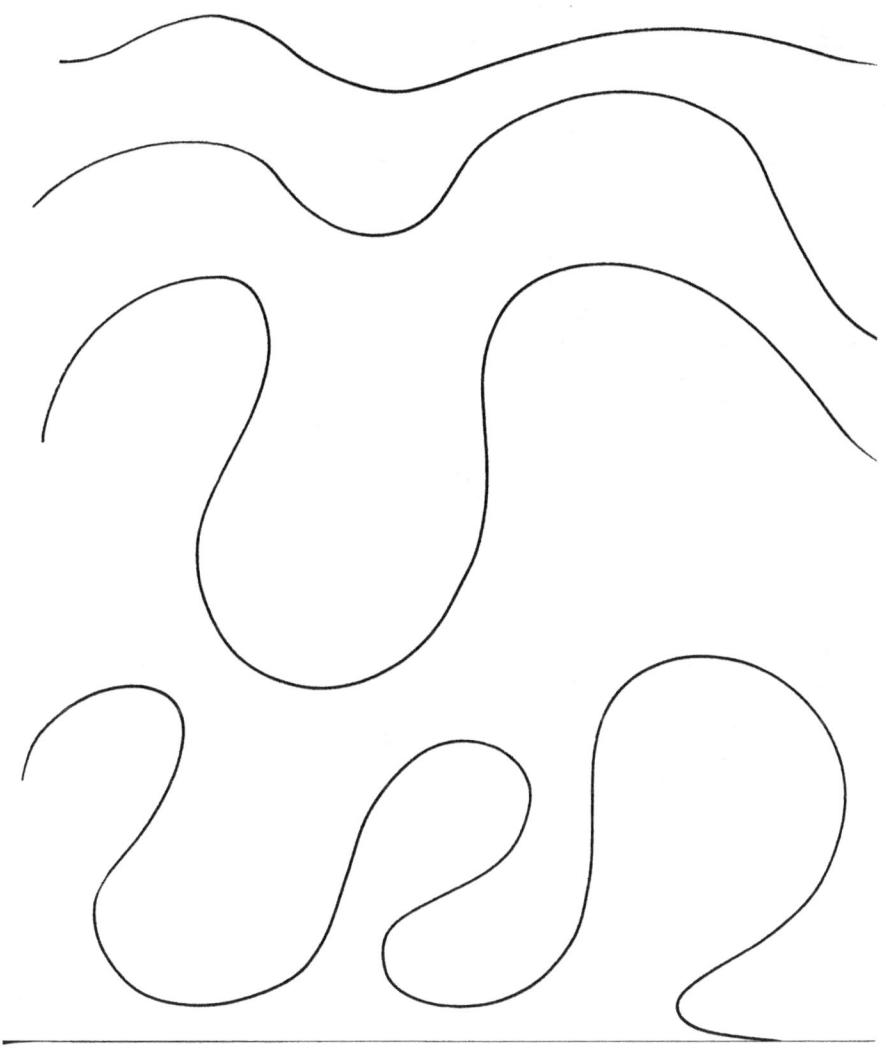

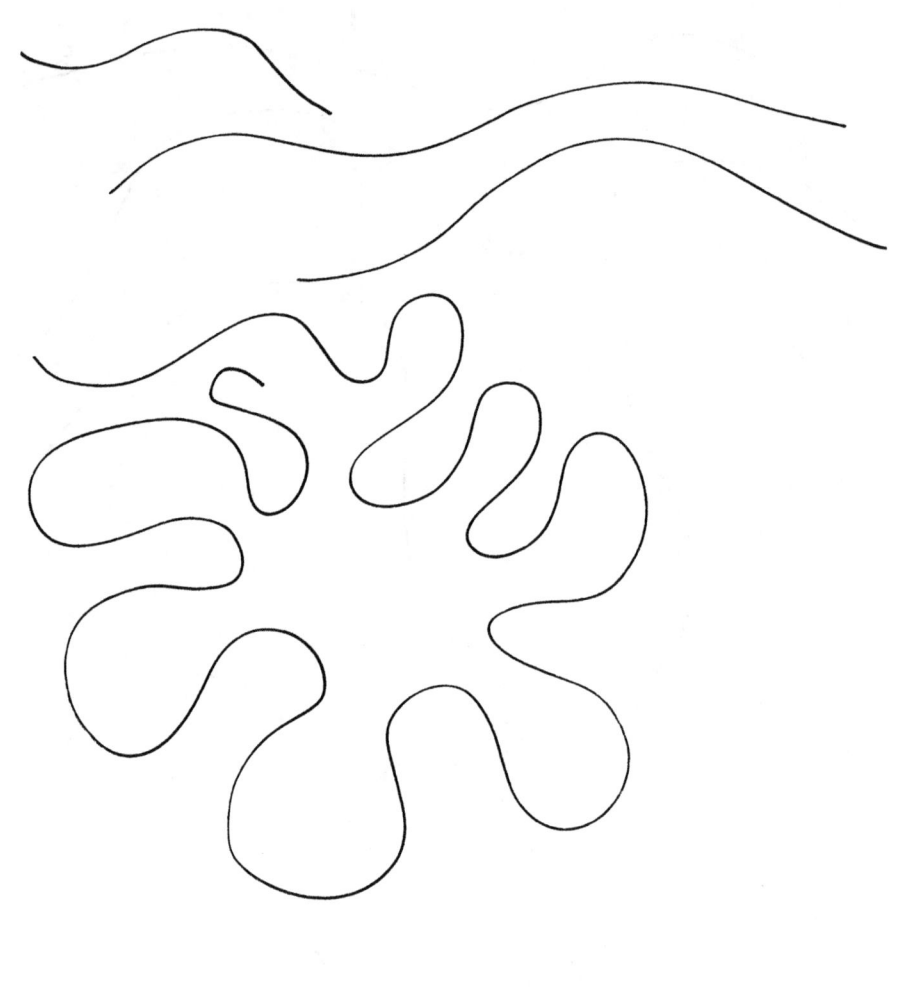

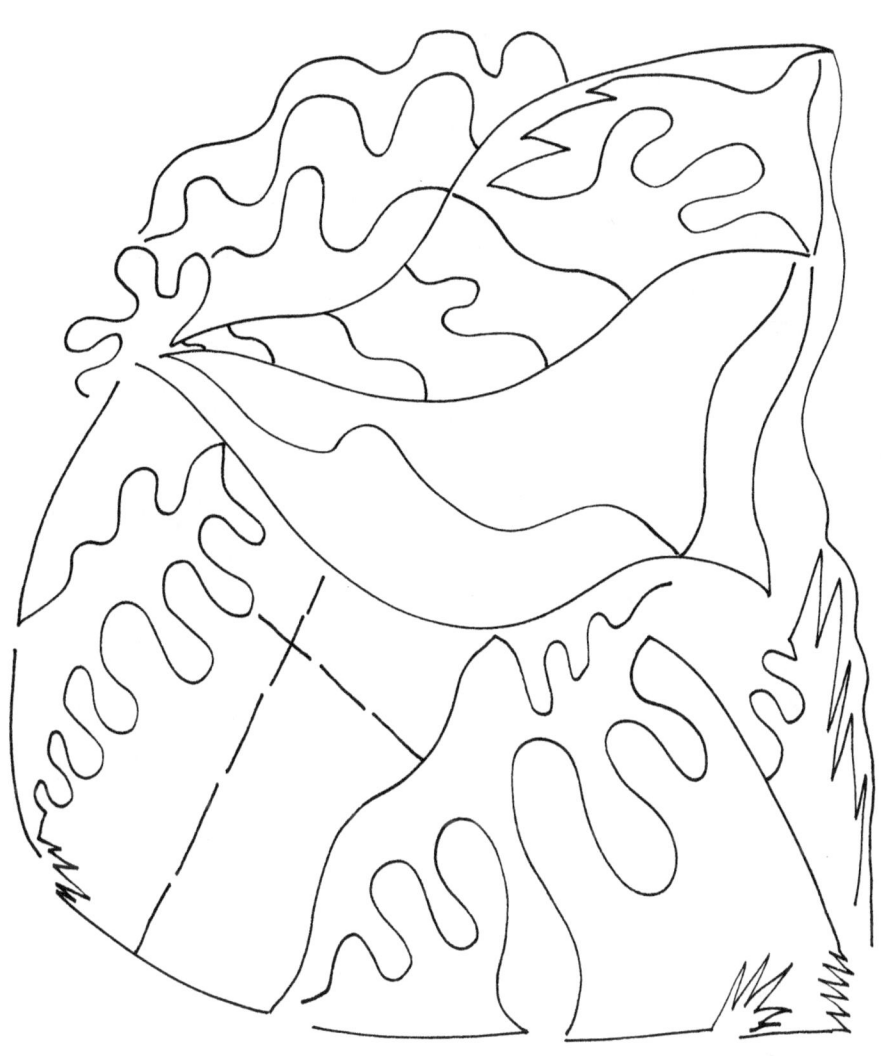

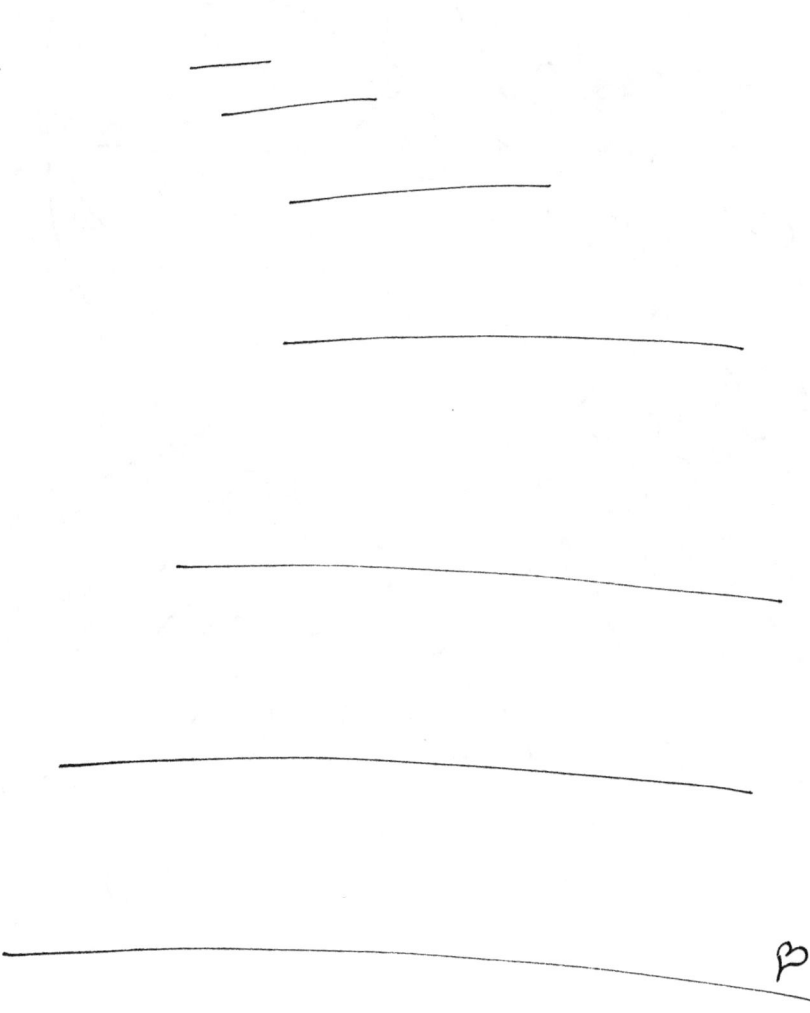

CONTINUES IN VOLUME 7

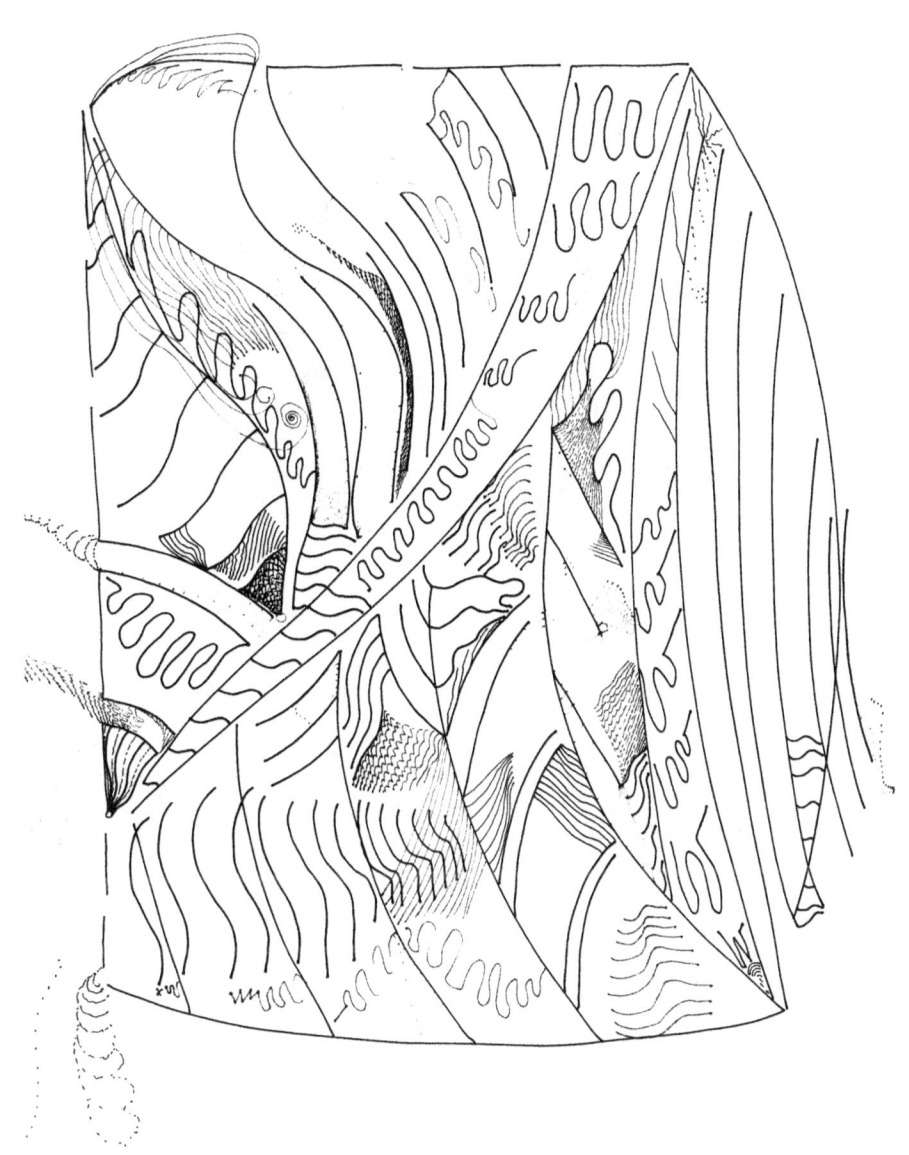